HYPERTENSION

Foods, Supplements & Medicinal Plants

Isabel M. Rivero

COPYRIGHT & CREDITS

HYPERTENSION Foods, Supplements & Medicinal Plants.
Copyright ©2017, 2024 Isabel M. Rivero
All rights reserved

Without limiting the rights reserved under copyright law, no part of this book may be reproduced, distributed, stored in a retrieval system, or transmitted in any form or by any means, whether electronic, mechanical, photocopying, recording, or otherwise, without prior written permission from the author.

Thank you for respecting this work. By supporting original publications and avoiding piracy, you help ensure the creation of new ebooks in the future. Your collaboration allows authors and publishers to continue bringing valuable content to readers.

Cover design: Desirée Mendoza M.
Photographs by Buntysmum and Cyberpunk via Pixabay

This book provides general information and is not a substitute for professional medical advice. Neither the publisher nor the author shall be held liable for any damages of any kind arising from the use of this content. Readers assume full responsibility for their decisions, actions, and outcomes.

This book is intended as a reference only and should never be used as a medical manual. Its purpose is to help readers make informed decisions about their health. It is not intended to replace any treatment prescribed by a doctor.

Original title: *Hipertensión. Alimentos y Plantas Medicinales* © 2017, Isabel M. Rivero. All Rights Reserved
© 2024 translated by Sara I. Afonso & Laura Mendoza

Prologue: A Guide to Wellness

Dear Readers,

Welcome to this journey toward better health! Since I began sharing my knowledge and experience, my primary motivation has been to make a positive contribution to your lives. That's why, through these pages, I aim to offer valuable information and practical resources that can genuinely help you feel better.

In this book, every piece of advice and remedy has been thoughtfully chosen for its proven effectiveness and practicality in everyday life. You will discover not only medicinal plants, supplements, and accessible foods but also detailed medical insights into this health concern, along with additional tips and answers to the most frequently asked questions–providing you with a practical, comprehensive, and trustworthy guide.

My goal is for this work to be your valuable and practical companion–a resource where you can find tangible tools to support you on your journey toward a healthier, more fulfilling life. Knowing that this work has a positive impact brings me great joy and motivates me to keep going. While writing requires effort, time, and perseverance, the knowledge that my books make a meaningful difference in your lives is my greatest reward.

Because your experiences are my greatest source of inspiration, I would love for you to write to me and share your progress. Feel free to share your progress by writing directly to me at **isabelmriveror@gmail.com**. Your stories inspire me and truly make my efforts worthwhile.

I sincerely hope this practical guide becomes your indispensable pillar on your journey to better health and well-being. Thank you for allowing me to be part of your life.

With love,

                        Isabel

INTRODUCTION

On our journey towards achieving optimal health, it's crucial to recognize one fundamental truth: no single "miracle" solution–be it a medication, herb, supplement, or food–can fully resolve an illness on its own. Solely focusing on managing symptoms, while neglecting the deeper "root cause," not only delays true healing but also increases the likelihood of recurrence. Instead, addressing the underlying cause of the problem can lead to a gradual reduction in symptoms and support genuine, long-lasting recovery.

You may have experienced times when treatments or medications didn't seem to deliver the results you had hoped for. This often occurs because restoring health requires a holistic approach–one that goes beyond surface-level treatment to target the root cause of the issue. Effective healing involves more than just the right therapies; it must also encompass vital changes. A well-rounded plan should include improvements to diet (the cornerstone of cellular health), enhanced sleep quality, better stress management, and the cultivation of healthier daily lifestyle habits. Together, these elements strengthen the body's resilience, boost confidence in recovery, and reinforce its natural ability to heal.

This book takes you on a journey through this integrative approach to health and recovery. In the first chapter, we'll provide you with accessible, straightforward explanations of the main causes behind this particular illness. Additionally, we'll cover its key symptoms, variations, early warning signs, potential complications, practical advice to manage them, and the essential medical tests necessary for an accurate diagnosis. This foundation sets the stage for understanding your condition and equips you with the tools needed to address it effectively.

As the chapters unfold, you'll discover practical, evidence-based strategies designed to support your recovery. These include detailed dietary recommendations, easy-to-follow meal plans tailored to your needs, and natural approaches such as supplements and herbal remedies that support gradual, sustained improvement. The guidance provided is both flexible and adaptable, allowing you to choose what works best for your unique health journey.

For those seeking a clear roadmap, the chapter titled **"Suggested Practical Plan"** serves as a comprehensive guide. This section consolidates the most important elements of recovery into an actionable framework, while also pointing you toward additional chapters for deeper insights and tailored advice. By using this plan as your foundation, you'll gain clarity and confidence in navigating the steps toward healing.

It's worth stressing that the guidance in this book is not based on subjective opinions or anecdotal evidence. Rather, every recommendation is supported by scientific research and validated by credible studies. To further reassure you, we've included a comprehensive list of references and studies at the end of the book. This ensures you can trust the methods and feel secure when implementing these strategies into your life.

Through a blend of understanding, practical tips, and scientifically-backed solutions, this book aims to empower you as you work toward true recovery and lasting wellness.

HYPERTENSION

Hypertension, or high blood pressure, might already be a part of your life, or it could be something you've recently been diagnosed with. Either way, you are not alone. Understanding it is the first step toward managing it effectively. More than just a medical term, hypertension is a challenge faced by millions every day, often without awareness until it has progressed significantly. Known as a "silent killer," hypertension can quietly advance over the years, showing little to no warning signs while gradually impacting vital organs like the heart, brain, and kidneys. Although this may sound concerning, it's important to remember there are steps you can take to regain control, improve your health, and lead a fulfilling life despite this condition.

At its core, blood pressure represents the force your blood exerts against the walls of your arteries as it circulates throughout your body, delivering oxygen and nutrients essential for life. While it may seem complex, blood pressure comes down to two key measurements: systolic pressure and diastolic pressure. Systolic pressure, the higher number, reflects the force when your heart contracts to pump blood. Diastolic pressure, the lower number, indicates the pressure when your heart rests between beats. A reading around 120/80 mmHg (millimeters of mercury) is considered normal, but when these numbers exceed this threshold consistently, hypertension becomes a concern. Chronically elevated blood pressure places strain on the cardiovascular system, silently posing risks to your heart, blood vessels, and other major organs.

Hypertension arises from multiple underlying factors that often interact invisibly, yet profoundly, within your body. A key variable is the resistance within your blood vessels, particularly the smaller peripheral arteries. This resistance depends on processes like vasoconstriction (narrowing blood vessels) and vasodilation (widening blood vessels), which are meticulously regulated by hormones, the nervous system, and chemical signals. Over time, disruptions caused by factors like stress, inactivity, an unhealthy diet, or genetic predisposition may upset this delicate balance, leading to persistently higher blood pressure.

Equally important is the concept of endothelial dysfunction, a critical mechanism behind hypertension. The endothelium–a thin inner layer of cells in your blood vessels–plays a vital role in maintaining vascular health. One of its primary functions is producing nitric oxide, a molecule that relaxes and dilates blood vessels, reducing resistance. When the endothelium becomes damaged or impaired, nitric oxide production diminishes. Without adequate nitric oxide, blood vessels remain constricted, increasing resistance and thus elevating blood pressure. This dysfunction often becomes a self-reinforcing cycle, placing additional strain on the cardiovascular system.

Another significant factor in hypertension is an overactive sympathetic nervous system, which regulates your body's stress response. Think of moments when you've felt acute stress: your heart races, and you feel heightened alertness. This is the sympathetic nervous system in action, releasing norepinephrine –a hormone that tightens blood vessels and raises your heart rate. While beneficial during short-term emergencies, chronic overactivation of this system leads to constant vasoconstriction and sustained high blood pressure. Over time, this increases the workload on your heart and arteries, amplifying the risks associated with hypertension.

What does all this mean for you? Hypertension may feel overwhelming, but it's vital to remember that every small step toward understanding and managing it brings you closer to better health. Knowledge truly is power. By gaining insight into factors like endothelial dysfunction, lifestyle habits, and stress, you equip yourself with the tools to take positive action. From nourishing your body with the right foods and supplements to adopting stress-reducing practices like mindfulness and exercise, even modest changes can yield significant benefits over time.

You don't have to face hypertension alone. Your healthcare team, loved ones, and the resources in this book are here to support and encourage you. Hypertension may be a part of your life, but it does not have to define it. Within these pages, you'll discover not only essential medical knowledge but also practical tips, complementary therapies, and strategies that empower you to take control of your health and well-being.

Let this book serve as your starting point–a chance to embrace a proactive mindset and transform your health. No matter where you are on your journey, there is always hope. Better health is within your reach, and this journey is one you don't have to take alone. Together, we'll explore practical steps for achieving a balanced and fulfilling life, empowering you to thrive despite hypertension.

Take this moment as a sign to move forward with confidence and optimism—because the best version of your story is waiting to unfold!

Types of Hypertension

Hypertension, or high blood pressure, can be categorized into several distinct types, each with unique causes, characteristics, and implications for health. Understanding these types is essential for identifying the most effective strategies to manage and treat the condition.

▸ **Primary Hypertension**: Also known as essential or idiopathic hypertension, this is the most common type, accounting for approximately 90-95% of all cases. In most instances, no specific cause can be identified for this type of hypertension; however, factors such as genetics, unhealthy lifestyle choices, and age may play a role.

▸ **Secondary Hypertension**: Unlike primary hypertension, secondary hypertension has an identifiable underlying cause, such as renal, hormonal, cardiac, or endocrine diseases. Treating the underlying condition can help control blood pressure.

▸ **Isolated Systolic Hypertension**: In this type of hypertension, the systolic blood pressure (the upper reading) is elevated, while the diastolic blood pressure (the lower reading) remains within the normal range. This condition is more common in older adults and may result from aging arteries and arterial stiffness.

▸ **Malignant Hypertension**: Also known as accelerated hypertension, this is a severe form of hypertension that progresses rapidly and can cause organ damage. It is characterized by extremely high blood pressure and may be associated with symptoms such as severe headache, blurred vision, nausea, and vomiting.

▸ **Gestational Hypertension**: This type of hypertension develops during pregnancy. It can affect both the mother and the fetus and typically resolves after delivery. If not properly managed, it can increase the risk of complications for both the mother and the baby.

‣ **Resistant Hypertension**: This refers to hypertension that is not adequately controlled despite the use of antihypertensive medications at maximal doses. It may be caused by factors such as non-compliance with treatment, excessive salt intake, untreated secondary conditions, or genetic factors.

‣ **Isolated Arterial Hypertension in Older Age**: This type of hypertension is characterized by increased systolic blood pressure in individuals over 65, while diastolic blood pressure remains normal. Arterial stiffness due to aging is one of the primary causes.

‣ **Renovascular Hypertension**: This condition occurs when there is a blockage or narrowing of the renal arteries, affecting blood flow to the kidneys. It may be due to polycystic kidney disease, renal arteritis, or renal artery stenosis. Treatment may involve surgical correction or dilation of the renal arteries.

‣ **Accelerated Malignant Hypertension** is an extreme form of hypertension characterized by a rapid and severe elevation in blood pressure. It can damage vital organs such as the heart, kidneys, and brain. This condition requires emergency medical attention and aggressive treatment to prevent serious complications.

‣ **Pulmonary Hypertension**: This condition involves elevated blood pressure in the pulmonary arteries. It may be caused by chronic lung diseases, such as chronic obstructive pulmonary disease (COPD), pulmonary fibrosis, or pulmonary embolism. Treatment may include medications to dilate the pulmonary blood vessels and improve heart function.

Causes

Hypertension, or high blood pressure, can be categorized into several distinct types, each with unique causes, characteristics, and implications for health. Understanding these types is essential for identifying the most effective strategies to manage and treat the condition.

‣ **Genetic Factors**: There is evidence that genetic predisposition may influence the development of high blood pressure. If you have a family history of hypertension, you may be at an increased risk of developing it.

- **Unhealthy Lifestyle**: Adopting an unhealthy lifestyle can significantly contribute to the development of hypertension. Factors such as a diet high in sodium (salt), low in potassium and nutrients, excessive alcohol consumption, lack of regular physical activity, smoking, and chronic stress can all increase the risk of hypertension.

- **Overweight and Obesity**: Excess weight, mainly when it accumulates around the waist (abdominal obesity), can raise blood pressure. This occurs because adipose tissue produces inflammatory substances that can negatively affect blood vessel function and fluid balance.

- **Excessive Salt Intake**: High dietary sodium (salt) intake can lead to fluid retention and increased blood pressure. Although individual sensitivity to sodium may vary, limiting salt intake to less than 2 grams daily is generally recommended.

- **Aging**: People are more likely to experience increased blood pressure as they age. This is partly due to age-related changes in artery elasticity and stiffness, which make it more difficult to maintain normal blood pressure.

- **Kidney Disease**: Kidney diseases, such as chronic kidney disease or disorders that affect blood flow and kidney function, may contribute to the development of hypertension. The kidneys are crucial in regulating blood pressure by controlling fluid and salt balance in the body.

- **Hormonal Problems**: Certain hormonal disorders, such as Cushing's syndrome, hypothyroidism, hyperthyroidism, and adrenal gland disorders, can increase the risk of hyper-tension.

- **Use of Certain Medications**: Some medications, such as oral contraceptives, nonsteroidal anti-inflammatory drugs (NSAIDs), steroids, and certain medications used to treat conditions like migraines, psoriasis, and cancer, can raise blood pressure.

- **Underlying Health Conditions**: Certain diseases and medical conditions, such as sleep apnea, diabetes, coronary artery disease, high cholesterol, autoimmune diseases, thyroid disorders, and cardiovascular diseases, may be associated with hypertension.

- **Environmental Factors**: Chronic exposure to environmental factors, such as air pollution, constant noise, and work-related or environmental stress, may contribute to the development of hypertension.

- **Chronic Stress**: Prolonged and chronic stress can lead to increased blood pressure. When stressed, our bodies produce stress hormones such as cortisol, which can temporarily elevate blood pressure. If stress becomes chronic, it can have a lasting impact on blood pressure.

- **Excessive Caffeine Consumption**: Caffeine is a stimulant that can temporarily raise blood pressure. Consuming large amounts of coffee, tea, energy drinks, or other caffeinated products can contribute to this increase.

- **Illicit Drug Use**: Some recreational drugs, such as cocaine and amphetamines, can rapidly elevate blood pressure. Additionally, chronic drug use can damage the cardiovascular system and increase the risk of developing hypertension.

- **Sleep Disorders**: Sleep apnea and related sleep disorders may contribute to the development of hypertension. Sleep apnea is characterized by repeated episodes of airway obstruction during sleep, which can disrupt oxygen flow and raise blood pressure.

- **Pregnancy**: Some women may develop hypertension during pregnancy, known as gestational hypertension. This condition may be temporary and resolve after delivery, but it can also increase the risk of developing chronic hypertension in the future.

- **Thyroid Problems**: Both hypothyroidism (low thyroid function) and hyperthyroidism (high thyroid function) can be associated with hypertension. An imbalanced thyroid can affect metabolism and circulation, increasing blood pressure.

- **Excessive Alcohol Consumption**: Excessive alcohol consumption can elevate blood pressure. Large amounts of alcohol can damage the heart and blood vessels and interfere with the effectiveness of blood pressure medications.

- **Blood Vessel Problems**: Certain diseases and disorders that affect the blood vessels may contribute to hypertension. These include arteriosclerosis, coronary artery disease, renal artery disease, and peripheral artery disease.

- **Endocrine Diseases**: Some endocrine disorders, such as

polycystic ovary syndrome (PCOS) and hyperparathyroidism, can increase the risk of hypertension. These conditions affect the body's hormonal balance and can alter blood pressure regulation.

‣ **Over-the-counter Medications**: Some over-the-counter medications, such as decongestants and nonsteroidal anti-inflammatory drugs (NSAIDs), can raise blood pressure. If you regularly take these medications, you must consult your doctor to assess their impact on your blood pressure.

Hypertension often arises from a complex interplay of genetic factors, unhealthy lifestyle choices, and underlying medical conditions. Together, these elements drive the development and progression of the disease.

Symptoms of High Blood Pressure

Hypertension, commonly known as "the silent killer," is a condition that often goes unnoticed because it typically presents no obvious symptoms. As a result, many individuals may live with elevated blood pressure for years without being aware of it, significantly increasing their risk of serious complications such as cardiovascular disease, strokes, or kidney damage.

In some instances, however, certain signs may indicate the presence of hypertension. It is important to emphasize that these symptoms can vary between individuals and depend on the severity of the condition. They are also frequently mistaken for other health issues. Some potential symptoms associated with high blood pressure include:

‣ **Headaches**: Headaches, especially at the back of the head, can be a symptom of hypertension. However, many other reasons can cause headaches, so they are not specific to hypertension. Headaches associated with hypertension are often described as throbbing and may be worse in the morning.

‣ **Dizziness and Vertigo**: Hypertension can cause dizziness and lightheadedness, which may result from high blood pressure affecting blood flow to the brain. However, it is essential to note that many other conditions can cause dizziness, so proper diagnosis is necessary.

‣ **Blurred Vision**: High blood pressure can affect the blood vessels in the eyes, leading to blurred vision or changes in vision. This can be a worrisome symptom and should be evaluated by a medical professional.

▸ **Heart Palpitations**: Some people with hypertension may experience heart palpitations, which are rapid or irregular heartbeats. This may result from the extra effort the heart must make to pump blood against high blood pressure.

▸ **Shortness of Breath**: Hypertension can affect the lungs and cause breathing difficulties. This can manifest as shortness of breath or difficulty breathing with physical activity or even at rest.

▸ **Fatigue and Weakness**: Some people with hypertension may experience generalized fatigue and weakness. This may occur because the heart has to work harder to pump blood through narrowed blood vessels, which can drain the body's energy.

▸ **Ringing in the Ears**: Ringing in the ears, known as tinnitus, can be a symptom of hypertension. High blood pressure can affect the blood vessels in the inner ear, causing constant or intermittent ringing.

▸ **Nosebleeds**: Some people with hypertension, especially extremely high blood pressure, may experience recurrent nosebleeds. High blood pressure can damage the small blood vessels in the nose, leading to bleeding.

▸ **Difficulty Falling Asleep or Insomnia**: Hypertension may be associated with problems falling asleep or staying asleep. This may result from the stress or anxiety caused by high blood pressure.

▸ **Chest Pain**: Some people may experience chest pain in severe cases of hypertension. This may be a sign of a more severe complication, such as heart disease, or an increased risk of a cardiovascular event, like a heart attack.

▸ **Concentration and Memory Problems**: High blood pressure can affect blood circulation in the brain, leading to difficulties in concentration and memory. Some people may need more mental clarity or help remembering information.

▸ **Swelling in the Extremities**: Hypertension can cause fluid retention, leading to swelling in the extremities, especially the ankles and feet. This is usually more evident at the end of the day.

It's important to remember that these symptoms are not specific to hypertension and may be related to other medical conditions. Additionally, many people can have hypertension without exhibiting any noticeable symptoms.

The most effective way to detect and manage hypertension is through regular blood pressure checks. If you experience any of these symptoms or have risk factors such as a family history of hypertension, obesity, diabetes, or smoking, it's vital to consult a healthcare professional for an accurate diagnosis and to prevent potential complications early on.

Possible Long-Term Complications

This section is designed to offer clear guidance and effectively highlight potential risks, with an emphasis on prevention. By doing so, you can take proactive steps to safeguard your well-being and minimize the likelihood of complications.

If not properly managed, high blood pressure can cause a range of serious complications that affect multiple systems in the body. The most commonly impacted organs include the heart, blood vessels, brain, kidneys, and other vital tissues, significantly increasing the risk of chronic diseases or medical emergencies. Some of the primary complications associated with hypertension are outlined below.

▸ **Cardiovascular Disease**: Hypertension is a significant risk factor for the development of cardiovascular diseases, such as coronary heart disease, congestive heart failure, myocardial infarction (heart attack), angina pectoris, and cardiac arrhythmias. High blood pressure can damage artery walls and promote plaque buildup, obstructing blood flow and increasing the risk of heart problems.

▸ **Stroke**: Hypertension is a significant risk factor for stroke. High blood pressure can weaken blood vessels in the brain, increasing the risk of rupture or blockage, which deprives the brain of oxygen and nutrients. This can result in an ischemic or hemorrhagic stroke, potentially causing permanent brain damage or even death.

▸ **Kidney Disease**: Chronic high blood pressure can damage the blood vessels in the kidneys, affecting their ability to filter waste and excess bodily fluids properly. This can lead to chronic kidney disease, kidney failure, and the need for dialysis or kidney transplantation.

▸ **Peripheral Artery Disease**: Hypertension can affect the blood vessels in the legs and arms, narrowing them and decreasing blood flow. This can result in peripheral artery disease, which is characterized by pain, cramping, and weakness in the extremities, and increases the risk of leg ulcers and amputation.

▸ **Eye Problems**: High blood pressure can affect the blood vessels in the eyes and damage the retina. This can lead to eye diseases such as hypertensive retinopathy, which can cause blurred vision, loss of central vision, and even blindness.

▸ **Dementia**: Uncontrolled hypertension over a prolonged period can increase the risk of vascular dementia. High blood pressure can damage blood vessels in the brain and reduce blood flow, potentially contributing to the development of dementia.

▸ **Sexual Problems**: Hypertension can affect sexual function in both men and women. In men, it can cause erectile dysfunction, while in women, it can decrease sexual desire and cause difficulty reaching orgasm.

▸ **Heart Failure**: Chronic hypertension can place additional strain on the heart, gradually weakening the heart muscle and leading to heart failure. In this condition, the heart cannot pump enough blood to meet the body's needs, resulting in fatigue, shortness of breath, swelling in the extremities, and other symptoms.

▸ **Aneurysm**: High blood pressure can weaken artery walls and lead to the formation of aneurysms, which are weakened, bulging areas in blood vessels. If an aneurysm ruptures, it can cause severe and potentially fatal internal bleeding.

▸ **Problems During Pregnancy**: Hypertension can increase the risk of complications during pregnancy, such as preeclampsia (a condition characterized by high blood pressure and damage to organs such as the liver and kidneys), premature delivery, and fetal growth restriction. These complications can jeopardize both the mother's and the baby's health.

▸ **Sleep Apnea**: Hypertension and sleep apnea are closely related. Sleep apnea is a disorder in which breathing is repeatedly interrupted during sleep, which can increase blood pressure. In turn, high blood pressure can worsen sleep apnea. This bidirectional relationship can increase the risk of cardiovascular disease and other complications.

▸ **Type 2 Diabetes**: Hypertension and type 2 diabetes often occur together. Insulin resistance, an underlying factor in type 2 diabetes, can also contribute to the development of hypertension. These two conditions can interact and increase the risk of severe health problems, such as cardiovascular disease and kidney disease.

▸ **Hypertensive Retinopathy**: High blood pressure can damage the small blood vessels in the retina, the light-sensitive tissue at the back of the eye. This can cause vision changes, such as blurred vision, decreased vision, and, in severe cases, even blindness.

▸ **Pulmonary Disease**: Pulmonary hypertension is when the blood pressure in the blood vessels connecting the lungs and heart is abnormally high. This can make it difficult for blood to flow and adequately oxygenate the body. It can also cause shortness of breath, fatigue, and, in severe cases, right-sided heart failure.

Reduction of Symptoms and Prevention

While hypertension can be dangerous if left uncontrolled, it is both manageable and preventable through lifestyle changes and healthy habits. Here are several strategies to help reduce symptoms and decrease the risk of developing it:

▸ **Adopt a Healthy Lifestyle**: One of the first and most important measures to reduce the symptoms of hypertension is to adopt a healthy lifestyle. This involves maintaining a healthy weight, following a balanced, low-sodium diet, engaging in regular physical activity, and avoiding excessive alcohol and tobacco consumption.

▸ **Follow a Proper Diet:** Diet plays a crucial role in managing hypertension. A diet rich in fruits, vegetables, whole grains, lean proteins, and low-fat dairy products is recommended. Additionally, it is essential to limit sodium intake, as excess sodium can increase blood pressure. A daily sodium intake of less than 2,300 milligrams (about one teaspoon of salt) is suggested. Furthermore, a diet rich in potassium, calcium, and magnesium can help lower blood pressure.

▸ **Engage in Regular Physical Activity**: Physical activity is another key component in preventing and managing hypertension. At least 150 minutes of moderate-intensity aerobic exercise or 75 minutes of high-intensity aerobic exercise per week, along with muscle-strengthening exercises twice a week, is recommended. Regular exercise helps strengthen the heart, improve blood circulation, and lower blood pressure.

Caution: Certain exercises and sports are not recommended for people with high blood pressure. You can find more details in the next section of this chapter.

▸ **Manage Stress and Practice Relaxation Techniques**: It is essential to manage stress and adopt relaxation techniques, such as meditation, deep breathing, or yoga. Chronic stress can contribute to increased blood pressure, so learning to manage it effectively is beneficial in reducing the symptoms of hypertension.

▸ **Follow-Up with a Physician Regularly**: Regular follow-up with a physician is another critical aspect of preventing and managing hypertension. It is essential to have regular blood pressure checks and follow medical recommendations. Sometimes, doctors prescribe medications to control blood pressure, which must be taken as directed.

▸ **Limit Alcohol Consumption**: Excessive alcohol consumption can increase blood pressure. Limiting consumption to moderate amounts is recommended, up to one drink per day for women and up to two drinks per day for men.

▸ **Control Your Caffeine Intake**: Caffeine can temporarily affect blood pressure. If you are sensitive to caffeine, consider limiting your coffee, tea, and other caffeine-containing beverages.

▸ **Get Enough Sleep**: Lack of sleep and poor-quality sleep can affect blood pressure. Try to get 7 to 8 hours of sleep per night and establish a regular sleep routine.

▸ **Reduce Stress**: Chronic stress can contribute to increased blood pressure. Find ways to reduce stress, such as practicing relaxing activities, spending time with loved ones, exercising regularly, and seeking emotional support when needed.

▸ **Avoid Tobacco Use**: Smoking or exposure to secondhand tobacco smoke increases the risk of hypertension and heart disease. If you are a smoker, seek help to quit. Also, avoid being around people who smoke.

▸ **Control Your Salt Intake**: Excessive salt intake can increase blood pressure, especially regarding table salt. Read food labels and avoid processed and canned foods, which are often high in sodium. Use spices and herbs to season your meals instead of salt.

▸ **Monitor Your Blood Pressure**: Share your blood pressure readings at home with your doctor. This can help you identify patterns and adjust your treatment plan if necessary.

▸ **Control Your Intake of Saturated and Trans Fats**: These fats raise blood cholesterol levels and contribute to hypertension. Limit consumption of fatty meats, full-fat dairy products, fried foods, and processed foods that contain trans fats.

▸ **Increase Your Intake of Foods Rich in Omega-3 Fatty Acids**: Omega-3 fatty acids in fatty fish such as salmon, sardines, and anchovies help lower blood pressure. If you don't eat fish, consider taking omega-3 supplements.

▸ **Control Your Blood Sugar Levels**: Hypertension and diabetes are closely related. Keeping blood sugar levels under control helps prevent and control hypertension. Eat a balanced diet, get regular physical activity, and manage diabetes.

▸ **Avoid Excessive Consumption of Sugary Drinks**: Sugary drinks, such as soft drinks and commercial juices, contribute to weight gain and hypertension. Opt for water, unsweetened tea, or herbal teas as healthier alternatives.

▸ **Reduce your Consumption of Processed Foods and Fast Foods.** These are often high in sodium, saturated fats, and trans fats, which raise blood pressure. Opt for fresh foods and prepare meals at home to control the ingredients.

▸ **Maintain a Healthy Weight**: Excess weight increases the risk of hypertension. If you are overweight or obese, losing even a small amount of weight can significantly lower your blood pressure.

‣ **Limit Your Intake of Medications That Can Raise Blood Pressure**: Some medications, such as nonsteroidal anti-inflammatory drugs (NSAIDs), decongestants, and oral contraceptives, can increase blood pressure. Talk to your doctor about your medicines and how they may affect your blood pressure.

Sports to Avoid with High Blood Pressure

For individuals with high blood pressure, it is crucial to take certain limitations into account when participating in sports, as some activities can increase the risk of complications. The most important contraindications to consider are listed below:

‣ **Isometric Exercises**: Activities that require sustained effort, such as heavy weight lifting or static exercises (e.g., planks), are not recommended. These exercises can cause sharp and sudden increases in blood pressure, significantly heightening the risk of adverse effects.

‣ **High-Intensity Sports**: Engaging in high-speed running, vigorous strength training, or competitive sports can lead to excessive blood pressure fluctuations. Such activities are not suitable as they can overburden the heart and vascular system.

‣ **Upper Body-Only Exercises**: Exercises focused solely on the arms or those requiring the arms to remain above heart level (e.g., boxing or overhead lifting) can significantly raise blood pressure. These activities should be minimized to ensure cardiovascular safety.

‣ **Contact Sports**: Intense contact sports, such as soccer, basketball, or boxing, may pose risks for individuals with moderate or severe hypertension. The combination of physical intensity and potential trauma–especially to vital organs such as the kidneys–makes these sports unsuitable.

‣ **Inverted Postures**: Activities that involve inversions, such as certain yoga poses or gymnastics, where the head is positioned below the level of the heart, can cause dangerous increases in blood pressure. Avoid these types of postures to minimize pressure spikes.

‣ **Sudden Positional Changes**: Abrupt transitions, such as quickly sitting up, standing, or lying down, can lead to blood pressure fluctuations. Such rapid changes can trigger symptoms like dizziness or fainting. It is recommended to make positional changes gradually and in a controlled manner.

It is crucial to remember that these recommendations may vary based on the severity of your hypertension and your doctor's specific guidance. Before beginning any exercise program or physical activity, consult your doctor. They can provide personalized advice tailored to your individual needs and medical conditions, ensuring your safety and well-being at all times.

Additional Remedies

In addition to the previously mentioned recommendations for managing hypertension, here are some other techniques that might be helpful for you:

▸ **Quick Trick to Reduce Tension**: Inhale and exhale slowly and deeply, only through the left nostril, for a few minutes. Cover your right nostril and keep your mouth closed.

▸ **Breathing Technique**: Sit comfortably with your back straight and close your eyes. You can also do this while lying on your back. Place the thumb of your right hand on your right nostril, letting your elbow point towards the floor to avoid tiring your shoulder. Keep your arm relaxed and place your left hand on your navel. Take a slow, deep breath through the left nostril, allowing your abdomen and chest to expand. Hold for a few seconds, then exhale slowly through the same nostril, completely emptying your lungs. Continue breathing through your nose only, in this case, on the left side. Repeat this technique 10 times.

▸ **Intermittent Fasting**: Another recommendation is to practice intermittent fasting, which involves consuming most of your caloric requirements quickly during the day and fasting for the remaining hours. For example, you can eat breakfast at 8 a.m., lunch at 1 p.m., and nothing until breakfast the next day. You can practice intermittent fasting twice a week and eat regularly on the other days.

▸ **Relaxation Techniques**: If you suspect that your hypertension may be related to stress, nervousness, fear, anger, or sadness, you can try relaxation techniques, breathing exercises, meditation, yoga, or EFT (Emotional Freedom Technique).

How to Measure Blood Pressure Accurately

Did you know that measuring your blood pressure correctly can significantly impact how well you manage hypertension? By following a few simple steps, you can obtain more accurate and reliable readings to support your health. Pay attention to these tips and prioritize your heart health!

▸ **Choose the Right Blood Pressure Monitor**
Always select a blood pressure monitor designed for use on the upper arm rather than a wrist monitor, as it provides much more reliable and accurate results.

▸ **Prepare Before Measuring Your Blood Pressure**
  ▸ Ensure you haven't eaten, consumed caffeine, or smoked in the last 30 minutes, as these activities can influence your blood pressure levels.
  ▸ Take at least 5 minutes to relax in a quiet, calm environment. This will help your body reach a true resting state.

▸ **Posture is Everything**
  ▸ Sit in a comfortable chair with your back supported and both feet flat on the floor, forming a 90-degree angle. Avoid crossing your legs.
  ▸ Rest the arm you'll use for the measurement (left if you're right-handed, right if you're left-handed) on a table, ensuring your forearm is relaxed and at heart level.

▸ **Position the Cuff Properly**
Make sure the blood pressure cuff is placed directly on your bare skin, with no clothing in between. If you're wearing a long-sleeved shirt or layered clothing, roll up your sleeves or remove any obstructions to ensure an accurate reading.

▸ **What to Do During the Measurement**
Remain completely still and silent while the reading is being taken. Any movement or talking can interfere with accuracy.

▸ **When and How Often to Measure**
For the most reliable results, follow these guidelines:
Take two consecutive readings during each session:
  ▸ Morning: Right after waking and after using the restroom.
  ▸ Before lunch: Before eating or taking any medication.
  ▸ Before dinner: Before your evening meal and any nighttime medications.
Wait at least 2 minutes between successive measurements to

ensure accuracy.

> **Record the Results**

Keep a detailed daily log of your readings, including the date, time, and specific measurements. This record serves as an invaluable resource for both you and your healthcare provider.

> **Verify Abnormal Measurements**

If your readings fall outside the normal range:
> - Take three additional readings, spacing each out by 3-5 minutes, and calculate the average.
> - Try measuring your blood pressure in different body positions, such as sitting versus lying down.
> - Monitor daily over the course of a week to identify consistent trends.

> **Consult If Something Seems Off**

It's not unusual for the first measurement to be higher due to anxiety or nervousness. This is why taking repeated readings is so important for obtaining an accurate average. However, if your blood pressure remains consistently high or falls outside normal levels, consult your doctor promptly.

Take Care of Yourself!

By measuring your blood pressure correctly, you're taking a simple yet powerful step to monitor and improve your health. Staying consistent and paying attention to your readings can help you stay in control and reduce potential risks.

Diagnostic Medical Tests

High blood pressure, commonly referred to as the "silent killer," demands early and accurate diagnosis to prevent serious complications. To achieve this, various medical diagnostic tests are available, designed not only to detect elevated blood pressure levels but also to evaluate the potential damage this condition may have caused to your organs and systems. The following are some of the most common and essential tests:

> **Blood Pressure Measurement**: This is the primary and fundamental test for diagnosing hypertension. A blood pressure cuff measures blood pressure in the upper and lower arms. Several measurements are taken at different times of the day to get a more complete picture of blood pressure values. A blood pressure reading of 130/80 mmHg or higher indicates hypertension.

‣ **Medical History and Physical Examination**: The doctor will review the patient's medical history, including any family history of hypertension and related diseases. A complete physical examination will be performed, paying particular attention to signs of damage to organs and systems, such as the heart, kidneys, and eyes.

‣ **Laboratory Tests**: Laboratory tests may be ordered to evaluate the function of specific organs and detect possible risk factors related to hypertension. These tests may include blood tests to measure glucose, cholesterol, and lipid levels, as well as creatinine and urea tests to assess kidney function.

‣ **Electrocardiogram (ECG)**: An ECG records the heart's electrical activity and can help detect possible cardiac abnormalities related to hypertension, such as left ventricular enlargement or arrhythmias.

‣ **Echocardiogram**: An echocardiogram uses ultrasound to image the heart and evaluate its structure and function. It can help identify enlargement of the left ventricle, abnormal heart valves, or blood flow problems.

‣ **Renal Ultrasound**: A renal ultrasound uses sound waves to obtain images of the kidneys and evaluate their structure and function. It can help detect possible abnormalities, such as narrowing of the renal arteries or cysts.

‣ **Stress Test**: The stress test evaluates the heart and circulatory system's response to exercise. It is performed on a treadmill or stationary bike while monitoring blood pressure and heart rate. This test can help identify possible limitations in exercise capacity related to hypertension.

‣ **Ambulatory Blood Pressure Monitoring (ABPM)**: ABPM is a test that records blood pressure over 24 hours while the person goes about normal daily activities. A portable device automatically measures blood pressure every 15-30 minutes. This test provides a more accurate picture of blood pressure values throughout the day and helps assess the effectiveness of treatment.

The selection of tests will be based on your individual clinical assessment and the associated risk factors.

Warning Signs

High blood pressure is often referred to as a "silent" condition because, in most cases, it does not present any obvious symptoms. However, when blood pressure reaches dangerous levels or complications start to develop, certain warning signs may appear. Identifying these symptoms early and taking prompt action can make a critical difference to your health. Stay alert to the signs and don't hesitate to seek medical attention if you notice them!

▸ **Severe and Persistent Headache**: Although a headache is not a specific symptom of hypertension, it can sometimes be a warning sign. If you experience a severe and persistent headache, especially if accompanied by blurred vision, dizziness, or confusion, seek medical attention immediately.

▸ **Chest Pain**: Chest pain can be a sign of severe complications of hypertension, such as coronary artery disease or angina pectoris. Suppose you experience a squeezing chest pain, tightness, or discomfort that radiates into your arms, neck, jaw, or back. In that case, it is essential to seek emergency medical attention, as it could indicate a heart attack.

▸ **Shortness of Breath**: Hypertension can affect the lungs and cause shortness of breath. You should seek medical attention immediately if you experience unexplained shortness of breath, especially during light activity or at rest.

▸ **Frequent Nosebleeds**: Frequent nosebleeds can be a sign of uncontrolled hypertension. If you have recurrent nosebleeds without an apparent cause, you should consult a physician to evaluate your blood pressure.

▸ **Blurred Vision or Vision Changes**: Hypertension can affect the blood vessels in the eyes and cause vision problems. If you experience blurred vision, sudden vision changes, loss of peripheral vision, or difficulty focusing, it is vital to seek medical attention immediately.

▸ **Extreme Fatigue or Weakness**: Uncontrolled hyper-tension can affect blood circulation and reduce the supply of oxygen and nutrients to tissues and organs, causing extreme fatigue and generalized weakness. If you experience unusual and persistent fatigue, even after adequate rest, it is essential to consult a physician.

‣ **Blood in the Urine**: High blood pressure can damage the blood vessels in the kidneys and cause bleeding in the urine. If you notice blood in your urine or changes in urine color, it is crucial to seek medical attention immediately.

Here are some of the warning signs associated with hypertension. If you experience any of these symptoms or any others that cause you concern, it is essential to seek immediate medical evaluation.

Warning Signs of a Heart Attack (Myocardial infarction)

It is crucial to recognize the early symptoms that may indicate a heart attack. If you experience any of the following signs, seek medical attention immediately:

‣ **Extreme fatigue** and difficulty breathing without an apparent cause.

‣ **Excessive cold sweating**, especially if it occurs suddenly and without explanation.

‣ **Chest pressure or discomfort**, accompanied by a sensation of heaviness or fullness.

‣ **Indigestion, nausea, or vomiting** without a clear cause.

‣ **Pain or discomfort in the center of the chest** that may persist for several minutes or occur intermittently. This can feel like uncomfortable pressure, tightness, or pain, ranging from mild to severe.

‣ **Pain or tightness radiating from the chest** to the shoulders, back, neck, arms, or abdomen, most commonly on the left side of the body.

‣ **Dizziness, difficulty breathing, nausea, or sweating**, accompanied by a generalized sense of discomfort.

Warning Signs of a Stroke (Cerebral Infarction)

Quick identification of stroke symptoms can save lives. Be alert to the following warning signs and act immediately if you notice any of them:

- **Sudden loss or weakness of vision,** particularly in one eye, although itSudden loss or weakness of vision, particularly in one eye, though it may also affect both.

- **Sudden weakness or numbness** in the face, arm, or leg, typically on one side of the body.

- **Sudden confusion,** difficulty speaking, understanding, or a complete inability to speak.

- **Difficulty walking,** often accompanied by dizziness, loss of balance, lack of coordination, or unexplained falls.

- **A severe and sudden headache** with no apparent cause.

What to Do If You Suspect a Stroke

If you observe any of these symptoms in someone, ask them to perform the following simple actions to evaluate their condition:

- **Smile**: Check if their smile is even or if one side of the face droops.

- **Raise both arms with their eyes closed**: Make sure both arms rise evenly.

- **Say their name or repeat a simple phrase**: Look for any slurred, unclear, or incoherent speech.

If the person struggles to complete any of these tasks, seek immediate medical attention at the nearest emergency center.

Important Note: Not all symptoms may appear in every case of a stroke or heart attack. Even if only one of the listed signs occurs, do not delay–seek urgent medical help right away. Every minute counts.

FREQUENTLY ASKED QUESTIONS

Navigating the intricate world of health can be a challenging experience, especially when faced with a diagnosis that impacts both your body and emotions. In such moments, many questions arise: What are the implications? What options are available? How will my daily life change? These and other concerns are common in situations like this. Here, you'll find practical and straightforward answers to help you make informed decisions with greater confidence.

This chapter is born out of a desire to provide support and clear tools to help you navigate this path with confidence. In an era overflowing with information–though not always reliable–it's crucial to distinguish between valuable insights and those that may create confusion. For this reason, I have compiled evidence-based answers to guide you through moments of uncertainty.

The question-and-answer format has been thoughtfully designed with practicality in mind, addressing the most common concerns faced by individuals and their families. The explanations are simple, concise, and focused on facilitating decisions that prioritize your well-being.

While the information presented here aims to be helpful, it is not a substitute for personalized medical advice. It's always essential to consult with your doctor to address specific issues that may arise.

Through these pages, I hope to offer tranquility, confidence, and steadfast support to help you face challenges with resilience. My goal is for this resource to inspire you and equip you with the tools needed to confidently confront this condition.

97 FAQs about Hypertension

1. What is hypertension?

Hypertension, or high blood pressure, is a condition in which the force of blood against the walls of the arteries is high enough to eventually cause health problems, such as heart disease.

2. What are the causes of hypertension?
The exact causes of hypertension are often not known but may include genetic factors, a diet high in salt, lack of physical activity, excessive alcohol consumption, stress, and obesity, among others.

3. What are the symptoms of hypertension?
Hypertension often has no apparent symptoms. For this reason, it is called "the silent killer". However, some people with hypertension may experience headaches, shortness of breath, or nosebleeds.

4. How is hypertension diagnosed?
Hypertension is diagnosed by measuring blood pressure with a sphygmomanometer. A reading of 130/80 mmHg or higher is considered hypertension.

5. What are the risks of not treating hypertension?
Not treating hypertension can increase the risk of severe health problems, including heart disease, stroke, kidney failure, artery damage, and eye damage, among others.

6. How can hypertension be prevented?
Prevention of hypertension includes maintaining a healthy weight, exercising regularly, following a healthy and balanced diet low in salt, limiting alcohol consumption, not smoking, and controlling stress.

7. Is hypertension a chronic condition?
Hypertension is usually a chronic condition that requires long-term management. With proper treatment, it is possible to control blood pressure and reduce the risk of complications.

8. What role do genetics play in hypertension?
Genetics can influence the risk of developing hypertension, as specific genetic variants affect how the body regulates blood pressure. However, diet and lifestyle play a crucial role.

9. What role does the nervous system play in blood pressure regulation?
The nervous system regulates blood pressure by controlling heart rate, the force of heart contraction, and the diameter of blood vessels through the sympathetic and parasympathetic nervous systems.

10. How can emotional stress influence blood pressure?
Emotional stress can temporarily increase blood pressure by activating the sympathetic nervous system and releasing stress hormones, such as adrenaline. These hormones can constrict blood vessels and increase heart rate. Stress management techniques like meditation and deep breathing can help mitigate this effect.

11. How does chronic stress affect blood pressure?
Chronic stress can raise blood pressure by activating the sympathetic nervous system and increasing the release of stress hormones, such as cortisol and adrenaline, which can constrict blood vessels. In addition, chronic stress can lead to behaviors that increase the risk of hypertension, such as unhealthy diet, smoking, or excessive alcohol consumption.

12. How can stress reduction help control blood pressure?
Stress reduction techniques, such as meditation, deep breathing, yoga, and regular exercise, can help lower blood pressure by reducing the body's response to stress.

13. Can children have hypertension?
Yes, although less common, children can also develop hypertension. This may be due to genetic factors, underlying health problems, or unhealthy lifestyle habits.

14. How does physical activity play a role in preventing hypertension in children?
Encouraging regular physical activity in children can help prevent the development of hypertension by improving cardiovascular health, controlling weight, and reducing stress.

15. What is primary hypertension?
Primary hypertension, essential hypertension, is high blood pressure without an identifiable underlying cause. It is the most common type of hypertension and usually develops gradually over time.

16. What is secondary hypertension?
Secondary hypertension is high blood pressure caused by another underlying medical condition, such as kidney disease, sleep apnea, hormonal disorders, or the use of certain medications. Unlike primary hypertension, which has no identifiable cause, secondary hypertension can be treated by addressing the underlying condition.

17. How does alcohol consumption affect blood pressure?

Excessive alcohol consumption often raises blood pressure by increasing sympathetic tone, disrupting electrolyte balance, and damaging the heart and blood vessels. Moderating alcohol consumption is essential to maintain healthy blood pressure and reduce the risk of cardiovascular complications.

18. Can caffeine affect hypertension?
Caffeine* can temporarily increase blood pressure in some people. However, the long-term effect of caffeine on hypertension is still under study, as it varies among people (*In the "Foods That Transform" chapter, we will discuss "Caffeine and Hypertension: Ally or Silent Enemy?").

19. What is the reference blood pressure, and how is it determined?
Reference blood pressure is a range considered normal based on population averages. Normal blood pressure is supposed to be less than 120/80 mmHg. It is determined through epidemiological studies and clinical guidelines.

20. What are the normal blood pressure ranges?
Normal blood pressure ranges are generally below 120/80 mmHg. Higher readings may indicate prehypertension or hypertension.

21. Is it possible to reverse hypertension?
While hypertension is often a chronic condition, it can be controlled and, in some cases, reversed through significant lifestyle changes and, when necessary, treatment with supplements, plants, or medications.

22. What is "white coat hypertension" or "white coat" hypertension?
White coat hypertension" is a phenomenon where a person has high blood pressure readings in the doctor's office but has regular readings in other settings. This may be caused by anxiety in the medical setting and does not always indicate an underlying problem.

23. What is a hypertensive crisis?
A hypertensive crisis is a medical emergency in which blood pressure reaches exceptionally high levels. It can cause organ damage and requires immediate treatment.

24. What is malignant hypertension?
Malignant hypertension is a severe form of hypertension in which blood pressure rises very quickly and can cause organ

damage. It requires urgent medical attention to lower blood pressure and prevent serious complications.

25. What treatment options are available for hypertension?
Treatment for hypertension may include lifestyle and dietary changes, supplements, antihypertensive medications, or a combination of these.

26. What is resistant hypertension, and how is it managed?
Resistant hypertension occurs when blood pressure remains high despite taking three or more antihypertensive medications. It may require a more intensive treatment approach, evaluation of possible underlying causes, and lifestyle and dietary changes.

27. How does cholesterol influence blood pressure?
High cholesterol can contribute to plaque buildup in the arteries, which narrows blood vessels and can increase blood pressure. Maintaining healthy cholesterol levels is vital for blood pressure control and cardiovascular health.

28. What effects does smoking have on blood pressure?
Smoking often increases blood pressure by damaging the walls of blood vessels, reducing their elasticity, and increasing heart rate. Quitting smoking can significantly improve cardiovascular health.

29. How does hypertension affect the brain?
Hypertension can increase the risk of stroke and vascular dementia by damaging blood vessels in the brain. It can also cause long-term cognitive problems.

30. What is metabolic syndrome, and its relationship to hypertension?
Metabolic syndrome is a group of conditions that occur together, such as hypertension, abdominal obesity, high blood sugar, and abnormal cholesterol levels. It increases the risk of heart disease, stroke and diabetes. Controlling blood pressure is crucial to managing metabolic syndrome.

31. How do insulin levels affect blood pressure?
Insulin regulates blood sugar, but it can also affect blood pressure. Insulin resistance can contribute to hypertension by increasing sodium and water retention in the body.

32. How does sugar consumption influence blood

pressure?

Excessive sugar consumption, especially in the form of sugary and sweetened beverages, often contributes to weight gain, insulin resistance, and, ultimately, hypertension. Reducing sugar and sweetener consumption is usually beneficial in controlling blood pressure.

33. Can weight loss help control hypertension?

Losing weight can significantly reduce blood pressure in overweight or obese people. Weight loss helps lower blood pressure by reducing the burden on the heart, improving blood vessel function, and reducing insulin and leptin levels, which affect blood pressure regulation. Even modest weight loss can have a positive impact.

34. How can weight reduction affect hypertension in adolescents?

Weight reduction can help lower blood pressure and improve cardiovascular health in overweight adolescents. Adopting healthy habits from an early age is crucial.

35. What is body mass index (BMI), and what is its relationship to hypertension?

BMI is a measure used to determine whether a person is at a healthy weight relative to height. A high BMI is usually associated with an increased risk of hypertension.

36. How does being overweight affect blood pressure?

Being overweight often increases blood pressure by forcing the heart to work harder to pump blood, contributing to insulin resistance and inflammation.

37. How does obesity affect blood pressure?

Obesity increases the risk of developing hypertension by contributing to insulin resistance, increasing sodium retention, and causing chronic inflammation. Weight loss often helps to lower blood pressure.

38. What are diuretics, and how do they affect blood pressure?

Diuretics, often called "water pills", help lower blood pressure by removing excess sodium and water from the body, which decreases blood volume and pressure on the arteries.

39. How does hypertension affect sex life?

Hypertension can affect sex life by causing erectile dysfunction in men and decreasing sexual desire in both sexes. In addition, some hypertension medications may have side effects related to sexual function.

40. What is pulse pressure, and why is it important?
Pulse pressure is the difference between systolic and diastolic blood pressure. A high pulse pressure can indicate arterial stiffness and an increased risk of cardiovascular disease.

41. What is systolic and diastolic blood pressure?
Systolic blood pressure (the top number in a reading) measures the pressure in the arteries when the heart beats. Diastolic blood pressure (the bottom number) measures the pressure in the arteries between beats. Both measurements are essential in assessing cardiovascular health.

42. What is isolated systolic hypertension?
Isolated systolic hypertension is when only the systolic pressure (the highest number in a blood pressure reading) is elevated, while the diastolic pressure remains normal. It is more common in older people and can increase the risk of cardiovascular disease.

43. What is diastolic blood pressure, and what is its importance?
Diastolic blood pressure is the pressure in the arteries when the heart rests between beats. It is essential because high diastolic pressure may increase the risk of damage to blood vessels and organs.

44. What is low diastolic blood pressure?
Low diastolic blood pressure, or diastolic hypotension, occurs when the pressure in the arteries between heartbeats is lower than usual. Dehydration, certain medications, or underlying diseases can cause it. Although it is often not dangerous, it can cause dizziness and fainting in some cases.

45. Can exercise help control hypertension?
Yes, regular exercise often helps lower blood pressure, improve heart health, regulate insulin, promote weight loss, and reduce stress, which are critical factors in managing hypertension. Activities such as walking, swimming, and bicycling are effective in controlling blood pressure. At least 150 minutes of moderate exercise per week is recommended.

46. How can aerobic exercise influence blood pressure?
Regular aerobic exercise, such as walking, swimming, or bicycling, can help lower blood pressure by improving the health

of the heart and blood vessels and by helping to control body weight.

47. How can resistance exercise affect blood pressure?
Resistance exercise, such as weight lifting, can temporarily increase blood pressure during the activity. However, when performed regularly and controlled, it can contribute to a reduction in resting blood pressure.

48. How can yoga help reduce blood pressure?
Yoga can help lower blood pressure by promoting relaxation, reducing stress, improving flexibility, and improving blood circulation. The postures, breathing, and meditation in yoga contribute to its beneficial effects.

49. How does sleep affect blood pressure?
Adequate sleep is essential for maintaining healthy blood pressure. Lack of sleep or poor quality sleep can increase the risk of hypertension by affecting hormone regulation and stress.

50. How does sleep apnea affect blood pressure?
Sleep apnea, a disorder in which breathing is interrupted during sleep, can increase blood pressure due to a lack of oxygen and stress on the cardiovascular system. Treatment, such as using CPAP devices, can help lower blood pressure.

51. What is arterial stiffness and its relationship to hypertension?
Arterial stiffness refers to the loss of elasticity in the arteries, which can increase blood pressure and the risk of cardio-vascular disease. Maintaining a healthy blood pressure can help prevent arterial stiffness. Factors such as aging and atherosclerosis may contribute to arterial stiffness.

52. What role does diet play in the management of hypertension?
Diet is crucial in managing hypertension. A diet rich in fruits, vegetables, whole grains, and low in salt and saturated fat usually helps lower blood pressure. The chapter "Foods That Transform" will discuss this in detail.

53. How can fiber intake influence blood pressure?
A fiber-rich diet can help lower blood pressure by improving heart health, controlling weight, and lowering cholesterol. Fiber-rich foods include fruits, vegetables, legumes, and whole grains.

54. What foods are recommended?

A diet rich in fruits, vegetables, whole grains, lean protein, and low in sodium* and saturated fat can help control hypertension. The DASH diet is an excellent example of a healthy eating plan for blood pressure.

55. What is the DASH diet, and how does it help blood pressure?

The DASH (Dietary Approaches to Stop Hypertension) diet is an eating plan designed to help lower blood pressure. It emphasizes fruits, vegetables, whole grains, and low-fat dairy products while limiting sodium, saturated fat, and sugar. The diet focuses on consuming potassium, calcium, and magnesium-rich foods and limits sodium and saturated fats.

56. How does the Mediterranean diet impact blood pressure?

The Mediterranean diet, rich in fruits, vegetables, whole grains, fish, and healthy fats such as olive oil, can help lower blood pressure by improving cardiovascular health and reducing inflammation.

57. How does hypertension affect the heart?

Hypertension can damage the heart by making it work harder to pump blood. This can lead to thickening of the heart muscle, coronary heart disease, heart failure, and other heart problems.

58. How can meditation help manage hypertension?

Meditation and other relaxation techniques can help reduce stress, which can help lower blood pressure. Incorporating these practices into your routine can be beneficial in managing hypertension.

59. How can meditation help control blood pressure?

Meditation and other relaxation techniques, such as mindfulness, can help lower blood pressure by promoting relaxation, reducing stress, and decreasing sympathetic nervous system activity. Regular practice of meditation techniques often has significant benefits for cardiovascular health.

60. How can deep breathing help control blood pressure?

Deep, slow breathing can help lower blood pressure by activating the parasympathetic nervous system, which promotes relaxation and slows the heart rate.

61. How can cognitive-behavioral therapy help control blood pressure?

Cognitive behavioral therapy (CBT) can help manage stress and anxiety, which are factors that can contribute to hyper-tension. People can learn strategies to reduce stress and improve mental and cardiovascular health through CBT.

62. What effect does magnesium have on blood pressure?
Magnesium helps regulate blood pressure by relaxing blood vessels and balancing electrolytes. Consuming supplements or foods rich in magnesium, such as nuts, seeds, and green leafy vegetables, is often beneficial for maintaining healthy blood pressure.

63. What role do the kidneys play in blood pressure regulation?
The kidneys help regulate blood pressure by controlling blood volume, electrolyte concentration, and the secretion of hormones that affect blood vessel constriction and sodium retention.

64. How does hypertension affect the kidneys?
Hypertension can damage the blood vessels in the kidneys, affecting their ability to properly filter wastes from the body. This can lead to chronic kidney disease or kidney failure.

65. What is renal perfusion pressure, and why is it important?
Renal perfusion pressure is necessary for the kidneys to filter blood properly. Maintaining adequate pressure is crucial for kidney function and the body's balance of fluids and electrolytes.

66. What is renovascular hypertension, and how is it treated?
Renovascular hypertension is a type of high blood pressure caused by the narrowing of the arteries that supply blood to the kidneys. It can be treated with medications, procedures to open blocked arteries, or surgery in severe cases.

67. How does aging affect blood pressure?
Aging can increase blood pressure due to stiffening arteries, hormonal changes, and decreased kidney function. Maintaining a healthy lifestyle is vital for controlling blood pressure, and it is also essential to monitor it regularly as one ages.

68. How can salt intake affect blood pressure?
Excessive salt intake can raise blood pressure by increasing blood volume and fluid retention, which puts more pressure on blood vessel walls.

69. How does sodium influence blood pressure?
Excessive sodium intake* can increase blood pressure by causing the body to retain more fluid, which increases blood volume and, thus, blood pressure.

70. How does potassium affect blood pressure?
Potassium helps balance sodium levels and relaxes blood vessel walls, lowering blood pressure. Bananas, oranges, spinach, and potatoes are rich in potassium.

71. Can potassium supplements help?
Potassium can help lower blood pressure by counteracting the effects of sodium. However, it is essential to consult a doctor before taking potassium supplements, as they are unsuitable for everyone. This is discussed in the "Supplements" chapter.

72. What is gestational hypertension, and how is it managed?
Gestational hypertension is high blood pressure that develops during pregnancy and resolves after delivery. It is managed with good nutrition, low-impact exercise (walking, swimming), regular monitoring, and, in some cases, supplements or medications safe for pregnancy.

73. Can pregnancy affect blood pressure?
Yes, some women may develop hypertension during pregnancy, a condition known as gestational hypertension or preeclampsia, which requires careful monitoring and management. Preeclampsia can be dangerous for both mother and baby. Pregnant women need to check their blood pressure regularly and see their physician.

74. Can hypertension affect vision?
Yes, uncontrolled hypertension can damage the blood vessels in the eyes, which can lead to vision problems.

75. What is nocturnal hypertension, and how is it diagnosed?
Nocturnal hypertension is elevated blood pressure during the night. It is diagnosed by ambulatory blood pressure monitoring, which records readings over 24 hours, including sleep.

76. What is ambulatory blood pressure, and why is it important?
Ambulatory blood pressure measurement involves continuous monitoring for 24 hours while a person goes about their daily activities. This provides a more accurate picture of blood

pressure levels daily and nightly.

77. What is the "nighttime blanket" effect on blood pressure?
The "night mantle" effect is the natural decrease in blood pressure during sleep. Lack of this decrease may be associated with an increased risk of cardiovascular events.

78. What role does calcium play in blood pressure control?
Calcium is essential for blood vessel contraction and relaxation. Adequate calcium intake can help keep blood pressure at healthy levels. Dairy products and green leafy vegetables are good sources of calcium.

79. What are calcium channel blockers?
Calcium channel blockers help lower blood pressure by relaxing and widening blood vessels, facilitating blood flow, and decreasing the heart's burden.

80. How can omega-3 consumption influence blood pressure?
Omega-3 fatty acids, found in fatty fish, some vegetable oils, and some supplements, can help lower blood pressure by reducing inflammation and improving the endothelial function of blood vessels.

81. How can intermittent fasting affect blood pressure?
Intermittent fasting may help lower blood pressure in some people by promoting weight loss and improving insulin sensitivity. However, the effects may vary between individuals.

82. How do hormones influence blood pressure regulation?
Hormones, such as adrenaline and aldosterone, play a crucial role in blood pressure regulation by affecting heart rate and the body's balance of fluids and electrolytes.

83. How does dehydration impact blood pressure?
Dehydration can temporarily decrease blood pressure due to a significant reduction in blood volume when changing position rapidly. However, chronic dehydration can increase blood pressure by activating compensatory mechanisms.

84. What is portal hypertension?
Portal hypertension is increased pressure in the portal vein, which transports blood from the intestine to the liver. It is

commonly caused by liver cirrhosis and can lead to severe complications.

85. How can folic acid influence blood pressure?

Folic acid, a B vitamin, can help lower blood pressure by improving endothelial function and reducing homocysteine, an amino acid that can damage blood vessels if elevated.

86. What is orthostatic hypotension, and how is it related to hypertension?

Orthostatic hypotension is a drop in blood pressure when standing up quickly, which can cause dizziness or fainting. Some people with hypertension may experience orthostatic hypotension as a side effect of medications. It may also be a sign of dehydration, heart problems, or neurological disorders.

87. How can apple cider vinegar affect blood pressure?

Some studies conclude that apple cider vinegar can help lower blood pressure by improving insulin sensitivity and reducing renin production, an enzyme that regulates blood pressure.

88. What is pulmonary hypertension?

Pulmonary hypertension is a type of high blood pressure that affects the arteries in the lungs and the right side of the heart. It can cause shortness of breath, fatigue, and, in severe cases, heart failure.

89. How can home monitoring devices help control blood pressure?

Home monitoring devices allow people to monitor their blood pressure regularly at home, which can help detect early changes and adjust blood pressure treatments.

90. How can acupuncture influence blood pressure?

Some research concludes that acupuncture may help lower blood pressure in some people by improving circulation and reducing stress, although more research is needed to fully understand its effects and mechanisms.

91. What is mean arterial pressure, and why is it important?

Mean arterial pressure (MAP) is an average value that represents the pressure in the arteries during a complete cardiac cycle. It is an essential indicator of blood perfusion to the body's vital tissues and organs.

92. What is coarctation of the aorta, and its relation to

blood pressure?
Coarctation of the aorta is a congenital condition characterized by narrowing the aorta. It can cause upper body hypertension and may require medical or surgical intervention.

93. What is central blood pressure, and why is it important?
Central blood pressure is the pressure in the main arteries near the heart, such as the aorta. It is a better predictor of cardiovascular risk than blood pressure measured in the arm, as it more directly reflects the load on the heart and vital organs.

94. What is oscillating blood pressure?
Oscillating blood pressure refers to significant fluctuations in blood pressure levels within a short period. It can indicate problems in blood pressure regulation and increase cardiovascular risk.

95. What role do beta-blockers play in blood pressure control?
Beta-blockers are medications that lower blood pressure by blocking the effects of adrenaline. They slow the heart rate and the strength of the heartbeat.

96. What is prehypertension, and how is it managed?
Prehypertension is a condition in which blood pressure is higher than usual but not high enough to be classified as hypertension. Lifestyle changes, such as a healthy diet and regular exercise, can manage it.

97. What is masked hypertension?
Masked hypertension occurs when a person has normal blood pressure in a clinical setting but high blood pressure elsewhere, such as at home. It may require ambulatory monitoring for accurate diagnosis.

SUGGESTED PRACTICAL PLAN

Living with hypertension can feel overwhelming, but it doesn't have to be. This guide is designed to empower you with simple, effective strategies to lower your blood pressure and reclaim your health. Packed with useful tips, this plan encourages small, meaningful steps that will make a big impact on your well-being–because every effort counts, and so do you!

▸ **Get to the Root Cause: Understand Your Hypertension**: When it comes to addressing hypertension, the first step is understanding what's causing it. Is it stress? Poor eating habits? A family history? Whatever the cause, pinpointing it is key to finding solutions. Explore these possibilities in the chapter "Hypertension", under the section "Causes", where we'll guide you in identifying triggers and taking steps to address or reduce them. Remember, recognizing the problem is the first step on the path to recovery.

▸ **Nutritional Supplements: Give Your Journey a Boost**: Sometimes, your body needs an extra helping hand. Nutritional supplements, when used wisely, can complement your efforts by accelerating progress and making results more noticeable. Find trusted recommendations in the next chapter to support your recovery and strengthen your health from the inside out.

▸ **The Power of Herbal Medicine**: Plants are nature's gift to us, and they're loaded with incredible benefits for managing hypertension. In the chapter "Medicinal Plants", you'll uncover tried-and-true natural recipes that gently but effectively lower blood pressure. These remedies, rooted in tradition, can work wonders in improving your overall health, one sip or spoonful at a time.

▸ **Nutrition: Your Ally in Every Bite**: What you eat matters, not just for managing blood pressure but for improving your overall quality of life. Certain foods are your best friends in this journey, while others should be minimized. Explore the chapters "Transformative Foods" and "Juices and Smoothies" for over 50 mouthwatering recipes tailored to support your health. Eating well doesn't have to be a chore—discover how delicious and fulfilling a hypertension-friendly diet can truly be!

▸ **Medications: Stay Informed and in Control**: If you're taking medication for any condition, it's crucial to monitor how your body responds closely. Certain treatments may worsen symptoms or cause unexpected side effects. Should this happen, contact your doctor right away to adjust your prescription or explore alternative options. Remember, your health comes first—never hesitate to advocate for yourself if something doesn't feel right.

▸ **Lifestyle Tweaks: Small Changes, Big Rewards**: Your daily habits play a huge role in managing hypertension. The chapter "Reduction of Symptoms and Prevention" provides practical, easy-to-follow advice to lower risks and keep blood pressure in check. Whether it's tweaking your routine or introducing healthier choices, these small, consistent steps can lead to life-changing results. You have more control than you think!

▸ **Move Your Body: Find Joy in Activity**: Exercise is a cornerstone of good health, and it doesn't have to feel like a chore. Even gentle activities, like walking or light stretching, can help reduce blood pressure and improve your mood. Love to dance? Great—turn up the music and move! Interested in relaxing exercises? Give yoga, tai chi, or swimming a try.
Before you start, take a look at the section "Sports to Avoid with High Blood Pressure" to discover which activities are safest for you. Remember, fun movement is the best kind of movement, and every little bit helps!

▸ **Manage Stress: The Invisible Trigger**: Stress is often called the "silent enemy" for a reason—it can sneak up on you and wreak havoc on blood pressure. That's why it's so important to make time for relaxation. Whether it's mindfulness, deep breathing, or quiet walks in nature, find ways that work for you to unwind and reset. Your mind and body will thank you for it.

Holistic Care for Coexisting Conditions

If you're also managing other conditions, like high cholesterol or diabetes, don't worry—you're not alone. This comprehensive plan can be seamlessly combined with my other specialized guides to ensure you're tackling every health challenge with confidence.

- **CHOLESTEROL**. Foods, Supplements and Medicinal Plants
- **DIABETES**. Foods, Supplements and Medicinal Plants

Through small but powerful changes, you can create a life that feels healthier, happier, and more in control. Let this guide be your roadmap to a better tomorrow. You've got this!

NUTRITIONAL SUPPLEMENTS

"True wealth is health" (Ralph Waldo Emerson)

Nutritional supplements have become a valuable ally in the pursuit of better health and an enhanced quality of life. These options–available in various user-friendly formats such as tablets, capsules, powders, or easily consumable liquids–are purposefully designed to complement your daily nutrition by delivering essential nutrients that can be challenging to obtain through regular meals alone. Packed with powerful components like vitamins, minerals, amino acids, antioxidants, and other bioactive compounds, these supplements are expertly formulated in precise proportions to meet the unique needs of every individual –even when the demands are high. Whether you're navigating restrictive diets, facing nutritional gaps, or coping with increased physical or mental demands, supplements can provide the extra support your body needs.

Beyond simply filling in nutritional gaps, supplements offer an array of tailored benefits to suit diverse lifestyles and health challenges. They can help boost energy, improve physical performance, support those managing fast-paced lives, and provide practical solutions for staying balanced and resilient. Their significance often becomes even more apparent during times of illness, specific health conditions, or chronic issues. In these situations, supplements do more than complement a diet– they can actively help restore altered functions, ease symptoms, and assist in more complex recovery processes. They serve as companions in the pursuit of health, helping you sustain and rebuild your vitality.

Effectively integrating supplements into your routine requires thoughtful use grounded in science and, when needed, professional guidance. By understanding their benefits and approaching them with care, supplements can evolve into powerful tools for improving your overall well-being in a sustainable and meaningful way. Remember–every step you take toward caring for your body is a step closer to feeling stronger, more energized, and more capable of facing life's challenges with confidence.

Take that step today. Your path to better health begins with small but impactful choices!

Essential Precautions

Understanding the risks associated with supplements is vital, as they can sometimes cause side effects, have contraindications, or interact with medications. It's important to thoroughly review the potential adverse effects detailed at the end of this chapter. Take a moment to assess your overall health and avoid any supplements that could conflict with the medications you're currently taking or exacerbate existing medical conditions. Prioritizing this step ensures a safer and more effective approach to improving your well-being.

Nutritional Supplements and Hypertension

Embarking on the path to a healthier life starts with understanding the undeniable connection between good nutrition and overall well-being. If you're managing hypertension, remember–you're not alone, and there is hope! With a few thoughtful changes and the right resources, you can take charge of your health and significantly enhance your quality of life. Nutritional supplements have become a dependable ally, helping you complement your diet while providing essential nutrients that support hypertension management.

This chapter is here to guide you, offering clear, practical, and easy-to-digest information about the most highly recommended nutritional supplements for addressing hypertension. You'll learn everything you need to know, including the suggested dosages, the correct way to take these supplements, the approximate time needed to see results, and the maximum period they can be used safely and effectively. For added convenience, all supplements are organized alphabetically, so you can quickly find exactly what you need.

Take a step toward better health today–your journey to managing hypertension starts here! With the right knowledge, making informed and meaningful choices about your well-being becomes easier than ever.

Coenzyme Q10

Coenzyme Q10, also known as CoQ10 or ubiquinone, is a

natural compound that plays a crucial role in producing energy in our cells. In addition to its energetic function, it has been the subject of research due to its benefits for hypertension.

▸ Coenzyme Q10 has been shown to have antioxidant and anti-inflammatory effects, which may help improve cardiovascular health and blood pressure regulation. Some studies conclude that supplementation with coenzyme Q10 may help reduce blood pressure levels in people with hypertension.

▸ Coenzyme Q10 has several beneficial effects on hypertension, such as improving endothelial function, reducing oxidative stress, and promoting blood vessel relaxation. These effects may contribute to lowering blood pressure and, ultimately, to managing hypertension.

Recommended Dosage:
The recommended dose is usually 100 to 250 mg per day.

Posology:
It is recommended to be taken preferably in the morning with breakfast to improve absorption.

Average Action Time:
The time to notice improvement can vary, but it usually occurs within weeks to months of continuous use.

Maximum Recommended Time of Continuous Use:
Continued use is generally considered safe for more than six months. Still, following a specialist's recommendations is essential to determine the appropriate duration for your needs.

L-Arginine

L-arginine is a semi-essential amino acid that plays a key role in several biological functions in the human body. It has been studied concerning hypertension because of its benefits for cardiovascular health and blood pressure regulation.

▸ It has been observed that L-arginine can improve endothelial function, i.e., the inner lining of blood vessels, which may contribute to reducing blood pressure. L-arginine is a precursor of nitric oxide (NO), a molecule that promotes the relaxation of blood vessels and helps regulate blood flow.

▸ L-arginine increases nitric oxide levels in the body, helping dilate blood vessels and improve circulation, resulting in lower blood pressure.

Recommended Dosage:
The recommended dose ranges from 3 to 7 grams per day.

Posology:
You should take it once or twice a day, preferably in the morning and/or before exercise. It can be taken on an empty stomach or with a small amount of food to facilitate absorption.

Average Action Time:
The time of onset of action may vary, but usually shows effect after a few weeks of continuous use.

Maximum Recommended Time of Continuous Use:
There is no established maximum time for continuous use, but it is recommended to stay within the recommended doses and consult a specialist if it is planned for more than six months.

Magnesium

Magnesium is an essential mineral that plays numerous roles in the human body, including regulating blood pressure. The role of magnesium in hypertension has been extensively researched, and its adequate intake can have significant benefits for managing high blood pressure.

▸ One of magnesium's primary benefits for hypertension is its ability to relax blood vessels. It acts as a vasodilator, which means that it helps widen blood vessels and improve blood flow. By promoting vessel dilation, magnesium can help reduce resistance to blood flow and thus lower blood pressure.

▸ In addition, magnesium plays a crucial role in regulating cardiac function and muscle contraction. An adequate level of magnesium in the body can help maintain a regular heart rhythm and prevent arrhythmias, which is especially relevant for hypertension.

Recommended Dosage:
The recommended dose ranges from 200 to 400 mg per day.

Posology:
It is recommended to take it once or twice daily, preferably in the evening before bedtime, to help relax muscles and promote

sleep. It can be taken with or without food. If a laxative effect is desired, it is best taken on an empty stomach.

Average Action Time:
The time of onset of action may vary, but usually shows effect after a few weeks of continuous use.

Maximum Recommended Time of Continuous Use:
There is no established maximum time, as magnesium is an essential mineral for the body. However, it is recommended to consult a specialist if it is planned to be used for more than six months in a row, particularly in individuals with renal or cardiac problems.

The Different Magnesium Compounds: The Most and the Least Laxative
Magnesium is an essential mineral with numerous benefits and plays various roles in body health. These include reducing pain, supporting muscle and nerve function, improving sleep, regulating blood pressure, and supporting the immune system. However, some magnesium compounds have laxative effects, which can be problematic for those prone to diarrhea.

Among the different types of magnesium supplements, magnesium citrate, magnesium chloride, and magnesium hydroxide (commonly found in antacids such as milk of magnesia) tend to have more pronounced laxative effects. These types of magnesium attract water to the intestine, which increases intestinal motility and may cause diarrhea in some people. These compounds can benefit individuals suffering from constipation, as they help make stools less dry and hard. The most laxative compound of the three is usually magnesium chloride.

In contrast, magnesium glycinate is a less laxative magnesium compound that may be more suitable for people with diarrhea.

Magnesium Glycinate: This compound combines magnesium with glycine, an amino acid. It is one of the best-tolerated forms of magnesium regarding gastrointestinal effects. Glycine is a stabilizing agent that can help minimize laxative effects and improve magnesium absorption.

As for the maximum recommended amount to avoid side effects such as diarrhea, it is essential to note that tolerance can vary widely among individuals. The recommended daily dose of magnesium varies according to age, gender, and other health conditions. It is advisable to start with low doses and gradually increase according to your tolerance.

Omega-3

Omega-3 fatty acids are essential fats found primarily in fatty fish such as salmon, mackerel, and sardines and in some plant sources such as walnuts and flaxseed. They have been widely studied for their numerous health benefits, including their potential for managing hypertension.

‣ Omega-3 fatty acids have been found to have vasodilatory effects. This means they can help dilate blood vessels and improve blood flow, decreasing vascular resistance and blood pressure.

‣ Omega-3 fatty acids also possess anti-inflammatory and antioxidant properties. Chronic inflammation and oxidative stress play a role in the development and progression of hypertension. Therefore, these effects are beneficial in reducing inflammation and oxidative stress in the cardiovascular system.

‣ It is important to note that omega-3 fatty acids are mainly found in natural foods, such as fatty fish, nuts, and seeds. However, they are also available as dietary supplements, such as fish or krill. If you choose to take omega-3 supplements, it is essential to select quality products and follow the dosage recommendations provided by the manufacturer or a health professional.

Recommended Dosage:
The recommended dosage ranges from 500 to 4,000 mg daily, depending on the product's concentration of EPA (eicosapentaenoic acid) and DHA (docosahexaenoic acid) and individual needs.

Posology:
Omega-3 supplements should be taken to facilitate absorption, preferably with a fat-containing meal. Depending on personal preference, they can be taken in the morning, afternoon, or evening.

Average Action Time:
The time of onset of action may vary, but the effect usually appears after a few weeks to a few months of continuous use.

Maximum Recommended Time of Continuous Use:
There is no established maximum time for continuous use. Suppose it is planned to be used for more than six months. In that case, it is recommended that you follow the manufacturer's instructions or consult a specialist, especially in individuals with coagulation disorders.

Potassium

Potassium is essential to the human body's fluid balance and cellular function. It has been extensively researched regarding hypertension due to its ability to regulate blood pressure and counteract the effects of sodium.

- Adequate potassium intake is associated with decreased blood pressure in individuals with hypertension. Potassium helps balance sodium levels in the body, which is vital for maintaining proper fluid balance and regulating blood pressure. Insufficient potassium intake and excess sodium contribute to the development and worsening of hyper-tension.

- Additionally, potassium can help relax blood vessels, improve circulation, and lower blood pressure. By dilating blood vessels, potassium reduces resistance to blood flow and promotes better cardiovascular function.

- Potassium is found in various foods, such as bananas, avocados, potatoes, spinach, beans, and dairy products. To ensure adequate intake, it is essential to include a variety of potassium-rich foods in the daily diet. However, potassium supplements may be considered if dietary potassium intake is insufficient.

Recommended dosage:
The recommended dosage varies according to individual needs but ranges from 200 to 4,000 mg daily.

Posology:
To facilitate absorption, potassium should be taken with meals or immediately after meals. It is essential to avoid taking it on an empty stomach to prevent possible gastric irritation. The dose can be divided into several intakes throughout the day.

Average action time:
Although the onset of action may vary, it usually affects electrolyte balance and muscle and nerve function within a few hours of ingestion.

Maximum recommended time of continuous use:
Continued use should be supervised by a specialist, as excess potassium in the body can be harmful, especially for individuals with kidney or heart problems. To avoid possible adverse effects, it is recommended that you follow your doctor's instructions and carry out periodic checks.

Vitamin C

Vitamin C, ascorbic acid, is essential to overall health and well-being. In addition to its known benefits for the immune system and skin, it has been investigated for hypertension and found to have positive effects on managing high blood pressure.

▸ One of its benefits is its ability to improve endothelial function. The endothelium is the inner layer of blood vessels and plays a key role in regulating blood pressure. Vitamin C helps maintain endothelial health and promotes the production of nitric oxide, a molecule that helps relax blood vessels and improve blood flow, thereby reducing blood pressure.

▸ Additionally, this vitamin acts as a potent antioxidant in the body. Antioxidants help neutralize free radicals, unstable molecules that can damage cells and contribute to chronic diseases, including hypertension. Vitamin C protects blood vessels and the cardiovascular system by reducing oxidative stress.

Recommended dosage:
The recommended dosage may vary depending on individual needs but ranges from 500 to 2,000 mg daily.

Posology:
Taking vitamin C, preferably during the day, with or without food, is recommended.

Average action time:
The onset of action may vary, but it usually shows effects after a few weeks of continuous use.

Maximum recommended time of continuous use:
Continued use at adequate doses is generally safe. If use is planned for more than six months, following the manufacturer's instructions or consulting a specialist is recommended, especially if adverse effects occur.

Vitamin D

It is a fat-soluble vitamin essential to bone health, the immune system, and muscle function. Beyond these benefits, its relationship to hypertension has also been investigated, revealing that vitamin D may positively affect managing high blood pressure.

One benefit of hypertension is its ability to regulate the renin-angiotensin-aldosterone system, which controls blood pressure and fluid balance. Vitamin D can help reduce renin production, an enzyme crucial to blood pressure regulation. This can help lower blood pressure and promote better cardiovascular health.

‣ Additionally, vitamin D has anti-inflammatory effects. Chronic inflammation is linked to the development and progression of hypertension. Vitamin D can help reduce levels of inflammatory markers in the body, improving cardiovascular health and lowering blood pressure.

‣ Vitamin D can be obtained through sun exposure and certain foods, such as fatty fish (salmon, mackerel, sardines), fortified dairy products, eggs, and mushrooms. However, supplementation may be necessary in some cases. When choosing vitamin D supplements, following a healthcare professional's dosage recommendations and considering any medications or medical conditions that may require restrictions on vitamin D intake is essential.

Recommended dosage:
The recommended dosage may vary depending on individual needs, sun exposure, and other factors, but generally ranges from 600 to 3,500 IU (international units) daily.

Posology:
It is recommended that people take vitamin D, preferably in the morning or during the day, with or without food. Vitamin D is best absorbed when taken with fat-containing foods.

Average action time:
The onset of action may vary, but it usually shows effects after a few weeks of continuous use. The response may vary depending on prior vitamin D deficiency.

Maximum recommended time of continuous use:
Continued use is safe at adequate doses. Periodic monitoring of blood vitamin D levels is recommended to adjust the dose if

necessary. Consult your physician if you plan to use it for more than 6 months or have any medical conditions that may affect vitamin D absorption.

Adverse Effects, Contraindications, and Interactions

Before incorporating the recommended supplements for hypertension into your routine, it's crucial to understand the potential risks involved. This section offers essential information about adverse effects, contraindications, and interactions with other medications or underlying health conditions. Taking the time to thoroughly review these details will empower you to make safe and well-informed decisions, always prioritizing your health above all else.

Coenzyme Q10

▸ **Side Effects**: It is generally considered safe and well-tolerated. Side effects are rare but may occasionally include stomach upset, diarrhea, nausea, or skin rashes.

▸ **Contraindications**: No significant contraindications have been identified.

▸ **Interactions**: Coenzyme Q10 may interact with certain medications, such as blood thinners, blood pressure medications, and chemotherapy drugs. If you are taking any medication, consult your doctor or pharmacist.

L-arginine

▸ **Side Effects**: L-arginine is generally safe when taken in adequate doses. However, high doses can cause stomach upset, diarrhea, and nausea.

▸ **Contraindications**: L-arginine should be avoided by people with certain health conditions, such as herpes, stomach ulcers, or liver disease.

▸ **Interactions**: There may be interactions with medications such as erection blockers, nitrates, and blood pressure medications. If you are taking any drugs, it is advisable to talk to your doctor before taking supplements.

Magnesium

▸ **Side Effects**: Magnesium is an essential mineral, and its supplementation is generally considered safe. However, high doses can cause diarrhea, stomach upset, and nausea.

▸ **Contraindications**: People with kidney problems should use caution when taking magnesium supplements.

▸ **Interactions**: Magnesium may interact with certain medications, such as antibiotics and blood pressure-lowering drugs.

Omega-3

▸ **Side Effects**: Omega-3 supplements, usually derived from fish oil, are well tolerated by most people. However, they may cause mild side effects such as a fishy taste, fishy belching, or stomach upset.

▸ **Contraindications**: Those with fish allergies should avoid these supplements.

▸ **Interactions**: Omega-3s may increase the risk of bleeding in people taking anticoagulants.

Potassium

▸ **Side Effects**: Potassium supplements may cause adverse effects such as stomach upset, nausea, diarrhea, or irregular heartbeat.

▸ **Contraindications**: People with kidney disease, heart problems, or those taking certain medications such as diuretics should use caution when taking these supplements.

▸ **Interactions**: The most relevant interaction is with certain blood pressure drugs. If you take any medication, you should talk to your doctor or pharmacist before taking potassium supplements.

Vitamin C

▸ **Side Effects:** Vitamin C is generally safe and well-tolerated in regular doses. Although side effects are uncommon, in high doses, they may include stomach upset, diarrhea, or heartburn.

▸ **Contraindications**: Individuals with certain conditions, such as kidney stones or G6PD deficiency, should avoid excessive vitamin C.

▸ **Interactions**: Vitamin C may interfere with certain medications, such as anticoagulants. If you take any medications, you should talk to your doctor or pharmacist before taking vitamin C supplements.

Vitamin D

▸ **Side Effects**: Vitamin D is generally safe in adequate doses. Although side effects are rare, excessive doses can cause elevated blood calcium levels, which can be harmful.

▸ **Contraindications**: People with certain conditions, such as hypercalcemia or sarcoidosis, should take Vitamin D supplements cautiously.

▸ **Interactions**: Vitamin D can interact with certain medications, such as glucocorticoids. If you take any medications, you should talk to your doctor or pharmacist before taking vitamin D supplements.

FOODS THAT TRANSFORM

"Every moment you eat or drink, you are either promoting disease or fighting it"

Throughout history, our diet has undergone profoundly radical changes, sharply diverging from the habits of our ancestors. Millions of years ago, early humans shaped their diet around what they could gather or hunt, relying on fresh and raw foods provided by their environment. The emergence of agriculture and livestock farming marked the beginning of a new era of human nutrition, further accelerated by the Industrial Revolution. However, it is important to recognize that while our dietary habits have evolved drastically, our genetics have remained virtually unchanged.

Over time, foods such as dairy products, grains, refined sugars, and vegetable oils were introduced, alongside the rise of intensive meat production. These innovations have made meals more accessible and convenient, yet they have also led to significant changes in nutritional composition. Furthermore, advances in food preservation and culinary techniques gave rise to new methods of storage and preparation, which inevitably impacted food quality.

In recent years, an alarming trend has surfaced: modern diets have become dominated by ultra-processed foods, contributing to the widespread increase in chronic illnesses. Conditions such as obesity, type 2 diabetes, hypertension, and a variety of cardiovascular and digestive disorders have all been closely linked to this dietary shift. Why is this happening? Primarily because ultra-processed foods are heavily laden with refined carbohydrates, unhealthy fats, added sugars, chemical additives, and low-quality vegetable oils. Even meats and other animal products from intensive farming systems are often filled with substances harmful to health. These processed foods have largely replaced traditional diets, which were built on fresh and natural ingredients, disrupting the equilibrium that once fostered optimal well-being among our ancestors.

Nonetheless, there is hope for reversing this trend: small yet thoughtful changes to our eating habits can have a significant impact on our health. Returning to a balanced, nutrient-rich way of eating, centered on fresh, whole foods, is essential for establishing a strong foundation for wellness. Integrating fruits, vegetables, root vegetables, legumes, nuts, and seeds into the diet is a powerful step toward revitalizing the way we nourish ourselves. Despite this, one major challenge persists: the consumption of these natural, unprocessed foods remains astonishingly low in many parts of the world.

Choosing a lifestyle rooted in mindful eating not only helps prevent diseases associated with poor dietary habits but also rejuvenates the body and mind. By prioritizing real, wholesome foods and cutting back on ultra-processed options, we can cultivate a healthier, more balanced, and fulfilling life. Now is the time to rediscover the transformative power of a healthy diet–not as a form of restriction, but as an act of self-care. Your health deserves that commitment!

Understanding the Link Between Nutrition and Health

How often have you asked yourself if what you eat truly supports your well-being? The relationship between nutrition and health is far deeper than we commonly realize. Understanding which foods promote wellness and which ones to avoid, tailored to your specific needs, is a powerful step toward improving your quality of life. This isn't a new concept; it has been examined and revered for centuries. Since ancient times, cultures around the world have recognized the therapeutic value of nutrition as a means to heal, strengthen, and sustain the body, leaving us a profound legacy of wisdom.

Traditional medical systems–such as Traditional Chinese Medicine, the practices of ancient Egypt, Greece, and Rome, Ayurveda in India, and indigenous healing methods across the Americas–delved into the restorative potential of natural foods. These practices emphasized the idea that food does much more than nourish; it can protect, alleviate discomfort, and even heal the body.

For many years, these age-old principles were often dismissed by conventional medicine as unscientific. Yet, modern research has gradually confirmed what our ancestors intuitively understood: the foods we eat directly affect not only our physical health but also our emotional well-being. Today, scientific studies continue to uncover compounds in food with therapeutic properties that help prevent diseases, reduce symptoms, and promote overall health.

Researchers have spent decades analyzing how certain foods strengthen the body and protect against chronic illnesses, identifying dietary patterns in populations with low disease rates that differ significantly from those in less healthy communities. These studies reveal the decisive role specific nutrients play in promoting vitality and longevity, with certain foods offering unique benefits such as anti-inflammatory properties to manage joint pain and chronic discomfort, antimicrobial effects to bolster immune defenses, anticoagulant actions to support cardio-vascular health, antihypertensive abilities to regulate blood pressure, and mood-enhancing compounds that alleviate anxiety while fostering emotional resilience.

What you choose to eat influences not only your daily energy but also your capacity to recover, fend off illness, and pursue a fulfilling life. On the flip side, a poor diet or reliance on unhealthy foods can exacerbate health problems, intensify symptoms, and undermine overall well-being.

The encouraging part? Every day offers the chance to make dietary choices that lead to better health. While external factors like pollution or environmental changes may remain out of your control, your diet is a fundamental tool for self-care. Each ingredient on your plate carries the potential to positively impact both your physical and mental health.

Learning which foods are best for your unique needs–and understanding which ones may harm your health–can empower you to find balance and achieve a healthier, more vibrant lifestyle. Nutrition, humanity's earliest form of medicine, is not just a pathway to wellness but also a connection to our roots, equipping us for a future filled with possibilities.

I invite you to explore how nutrition can become your strongest ally in easing ailments, building resilience, and fostering happiness. Are you ready to embrace this journey of discovery and transformation? Your well-being is within your control, and every meal is a chance to create a life of greater health and vitality.

Start today: Nourish your body, refresh your mind, and live fully.

Cooking Techniques

Healthy cooking is essential for everyone, especially after the age of 40. Below are various cooking techniques along with their related health benefits and potential risks.

Healthier Ways of Cooking

▸ **Steaming**: Steaming is an excellent method for preserving nutrients, as it does not require the use of additional fats. It helps keep food tender and juicy while being a gentle cooking technique that does not contribute to the formation of harmful compounds.

▸ **Oven roasting**: Oven roasting is a healthy option that does not require added oils. Foods like vegetables, fish, and chicken can be roasted in the oven to create nutritious and flavorful meals.

▸ **Light sautéing**: This method involves quickly cooking food over high heat with a small amount of healthy oil, such as olive or coconut oil. Light sautéing helps maintain the food's texture and nutrients while cooking it efficiently.

▸ **Boiling**: Boiling is a healthy cooking method, particularly for vegetables. It preserves nutrients and creates a tender texture. However, it is crucial to avoid overcooking to minimize nutrient loss.

▸ **Baking**: Baking is an excellent way to prepare food without the need for added oils. Foods like fish, poultry, vegetables, and whole grains can be baked for healthy and flavorful dishes.

Less Healthy Ways of Cooking

▸ **Frying**: Frying involves submerging food in hot oil, which significantly increases its saturated fat and calorie content. Additionally, frying at high temperatures can produce harmful compounds that pose health risks.

▸ **Breading and battering**: Coating food in breading or batter increases its calorie and fat content. These coatings can absorb more oil during cooking, resulting in a less nutritious meal.

▸ **Creamy sauces and dressings**: Cream-based sauces and

dressings often contain high levels of saturated fat and excess calories. These can contribute to inflammation and exacerbate pain.

▸ **Grilling at high temperatures**: Cooking food on the grill at high heat can generate harmful compounds, such as polycyclic aromatic hydrocarbons (PAHs) and heterocyclic amines (HCAs), which have been associated with an increased cancer risk. Additionally, grilled meats can produce inflammatory substances.

Remember, the way you cook food significantly impacts its nutritional value and its overall effects on your health. Choosing healthy cooking methods ensures you maximize the benefits of your meals while reducing potential negative effects.

Healing Foods According to TCM

The wisdom of Traditional Chinese Medicine (TCM), with centuries of practice, emphasizes a variety of foods that can naturally help regulate blood pressure. Below, they are organized alphabetically for easy reference:

Apple (Malus pumila)

A popular and healthy fruit, a simple recipe involves eating 1 or 2 apples on an empty stomach twice daily, morning and evening. Alternatively, extract the juice from the apples and drink 100 ml thrice daily for 10 days. However, according to Traditional Chinese Medicine, excessive consumption of apples may cause abdominal bloating due to their fresh nature, so moderation is recommended.

Bean (Vicia faba)

Fresh flowers (or smaller quantities of dried flowers) can be cooked and consumed to leverage the benefits of fava beans in regulating blood pressure. It is important to note that, according to TCM, excessive consumption can cause abdominal bloating. Additionally, some individuals may develop favism or "fava bean sickness" after consuming fava beans. Symptoms include dark urine, jaundice, fever, malaise, and vomiting. If these symptoms occur, seek medical attention immediately. This hereditary disease warrants extra precautions for those with a family history of favism.

Celery (Apium graveolens)

Celery can also be beneficial in regulating blood pressure. There are different ways to consume it:

You can extract the juice from a good amount of washed and crushed celery and drink 300 ml twice daily.
Prepare an infusion by boiling and consuming 500 grams of celery with brown sugar.
Another option is to boil 250 grams of celery with 10 red dates in a saucepan with water. Then, drink the liquid and eat the dates.
You can wash 250 grams of fresh celery (or 100 grams of dried celery), boil it for 2 minutes, chop it, and extract its juice. Then, you can drink the juice twice a day.

Corn (Zea mays)

A versatile food with various uses, a simple recipe involves boiling 30 grams of corn stigmas in 1 liter of water until reduced to 500 ml and drinking it on an empty stomach. Another option is to prepare a broth with 30 grams of corn stigmas, 100 grams of watermelon rind, and 50 grams of banana peel. Precautions are essential when consuming corn. According to Traditional Chinese Medicine, moldy corn can produce carcinogenic substances such as "Aspergillus flavus", so avoid eating moldy or spoiled corn.

Cucumber (Cucumis sativus)

Dried cucumber shoots can be used to prepare a decoction, which should be consumed in three daily doses to benefit from the cucumber's ability to regulate blood pressure. However, according to Traditional Chinese Medicine, individuals with pulmonary or stomach insufficiency or cold should consume cucumber in small quantities to avoid cough, diarrhea, or enteritis due to its cold nature. Additionally, if consumed raw, special care should be taken with hygiene to prevent the entry of pathogenic germs through the mouth.

Garlic (Allium sativum)

One recipe for maximizing garlic's benefits is to prepare a mixture of 30 large garlic cloves, brown sugar, and vinegar. Clean the garlic well and then mix it with the vinegar and sugar. After a week, the garlic will have a sweet and sour taste. You should eat 2 cloves of garlic on an empty stomach, accompanied by a few sips of the liquid. Generally, within 10-15 days, blood pressure tends to normalize.

However, according to Traditional Chinese Medicine, garlic should not be eaten in excess for a long time (more than 3 months), as it can increase internal heat and affect eyesight. It is also not advisable to abuse garlic for those who suffer from stomach dysfunctions.

Grape (Vitis vinifera)

To regulate blood pressure, prepare a grape and celery juice mixture and take it two to three times daily. However, be cautious about excessive grape consumption, as their high sugar content can cause diarrhea, restlessness, and drowsiness. Consuming grapes in moderation is essential to avoid these adverse effects.

Groundnut (Arachis hypogea)

Several recipes can be followed to benefit from peanuts in regulating blood pressure. One option is to cook peanut shells and consume the preparation once a day. Another recipe involves macerating red-skinned peanuts in rice vinegar for 10 days and then consuming 10 peanuts twice a day over a prolonged period. However, it is essential to note that, according to Traditional Chinese Medicine, people suffering from diarrhea should not consume peanuts due to their high-fat content, as they can lubricate the intestine and worsen symptoms.

Kiwifruit (Actinidia chinensis)

This delicious and nutritious fruit can be enjoyed in various ways. A simple recipe is to eat 30 grams of fresh peeled kiwi 2 or 3 times a day. Alternatively, 50 grams of dried kiwi can be boiled in water and taken once a day. However, caution is advised when consuming kiwifruit. According to Traditional Chinese Medicine, its cold nature can cause diarrhea and should not be overeaten, especially by individuals predisposed to diarrhea or with a sensitive stomach.

Lemon (Citrus limon)

Known for its rich flavor and health benefits, a simple recipe involves taking fresh lemon slices and brown sugar, storing them for a month, and then consuming the prepared slices as an infusion (5 slices, 1 or 2 times a day). However, precautions are necessary. According to Traditional Chinese Medicine, those suffering from gastroduodenal ulcers or hyperchlorhydria should avoid lemon juice due to its high citric acid content.

Melon (Cucumis melo)

To benefit from melon's ability to regulate blood pressure, dried stems of melon, cucumber, and watermelon can be used to prepare a decoction. Boil them in 500 ml of water until reduced to 100 ml and consume 1 or 2 times daily for a month. However, according to Traditional Chinese Medicine, due to its cold nature, melon should not be consumed by individuals with stomach or intestinal weakness due to cold factors or those suffering from diarrhea. Caution is also advised with the stalk of the melon, as it is toxic and should only be consumed in specific doses to induce vomiting. Additionally, those suffering from hemorrhages or asthenia should be cautious when consuming melon.

Mung Bean (Phaseolus radiatus)

To utilize the benefits of mung beans in regulating blood pressure, boil 100 grams of mung beans with 50 grams of seaweed until well-cooked. It is recommended to consume it with a little crystallized sugar. Besides regulating blood pressure, this recipe may also help reduce excess fat in the blood. However, due to its cold nature, people with spleen or stomach weakness should consume it in moderation, according to Traditional Chinese Medicine.

Onion (Allium cepa)

Onions can be consumed regularly as part of the daily diet to take advantage of their benefits in regulating blood pressure. No specific precautions are mentioned in relation to Traditional Chinese Medicine.

Pea (Pisum sativum)

Tender pea shoots can benefit from the pea's ability to regulate blood pressure. Crush the sprouts to extract the juice, which can be consumed in 200 ml portions twice daily. The juice can also be slightly warmed before drinking. However, according to Traditional Chinese Medicine, it should not be consumed excessively, as it may cause flatulence.

Persimmon (Diospyros kaki)

Persimmon can also be beneficial in regulating blood pressure.

Various recipes can be followed, such as extracting persimmon juice and mixing it with cow's milk or rice broth to be consumed urgently or when symptoms of apoplexy occur. Another option is to cook dried persimmons and consume them twice daily. You can squeeze green persimmons and drink 100 ml of juice twice or thrice daily. However, it is essential to remember that, according to Traditional Chinese Medicine, persimmons should not be consumed on an empty stomach, nor should unripe persimmons be eaten. It is not recommended for people with weak spleen or stomach energy, diarrhea, colds, flu, or an unhealthy constitution. Consuming persimmon should also be avoided at the same time as vinegar or crab, as this can cause intestinal obstruction and digestive symptoms.

Plantain (Musa paradisiaca)

To harness the benefits of plantain in regulating blood pressure, consume 1 or 2 plantains, 2 to 3 times a day, for an indefinite period. You can also use plantain skins to prepare various recipes, such as cooking them and drinking the broth as an infusion, accompanied by the plantain flesh. However, according to Traditional Chinese Medicine, individuals with spleen or stomach weakness, stomach pains, or diarrhea should consume plantains in small quantities due to their cold nature. Those suffering from reflux or heartburn should completely abstain from consuming plantain.

Sesame (Sesamum indicum)

To capitalize on sesame's benefits, prepare a mixture of sesame, vinegar, honey, and brown-shell egg white. This mixture should be consumed over two days, 3 times daily, and is considered effective if taken frequently. However, caution is advised when consuming sesame due to its high oil content, which can act as a lubricant and have a laxative effect, making it helpful for constipation. However, individuals suffering from diarrhea should be cautious. Additionally, moldy sesame is toxic and should not be consumed, and the remains of sesame after oil extraction should not be used as animal feed due to their toxicity.

Spinach (Spinacia oleracea):

To benefit from spinach's ability to regulate blood pressure, spinach can be washed well and then cooked briefly in boiling water. It is recommended to consume them with sesame oil on top. However, it is essential to remember that, according to Traditional Chinese Medicine, people suffering from stomach problems or diarrhea should consume spinach in limited quantities due to its cold and lubricating nature. Additionally, spinach contains oxalic acid, so drinking it with calcium-rich foods is not recommended, as it hinders calcium absorption and digestion.

Sunflower (Helianthus annuus)

To benefit from sunflower seeds regulating blood pressure, peel and consume sunflower seeds, and drink celery juice. This combination should be performed twice daily, morning and evening, for a month. However, according to Traditional Chinese Medicine, people with very loose or liquid stools and digestive problems should consume sunflower in limited amounts due to its high fat content, which can have lubricating and laxative properties. In addition, when sunflower oil is used for cooking, it should not be overheated.

Sweet Potato (Ipomoea batatas)

Sweet potatoes can also be beneficial in regulating blood pressure. One way to consume it is to prepare a rice soup by mixing 250 grams of washed and chopped sweet potato with 150 grams of basmati rice. Take this soup in two daily doses.

Remember that these are just a few examples of how to consume celery and sweet potatoes. It is essential to remember the precautions and limitations mentioned above.

Tropical Pineapple (Ananas comosus)

Peel the pineapple and extract its juice to benefit from its ability to regulate blood pressure. Take 30 ml mixed with cold water 2 to 3 times daily. However, according to Traditional Chinese Medicine, due to its glycoside and bromelain content, some individuals may experience allergic reactions or irritation of the oral mucosa when consuming pineapple. Therefore, macerating the pulp in salt water before consumption is recommended to avoid these reactions. Additionally, people suffering from digestive ulcers, coagulation problems, or severe liver or kidney ailments should avoid excessive consumption of pineapple.

Hypertension during Pregnancy
Soybeans (Glycine max)

To leverage the benefits of soybeans, use bean sprouts and cook them for 3 to 4 hours to obtain a warm broth. This broth can be consumed. However, caution is necessary when consuming soy in excess, as it can cause gas accumulation and bloating. Soy also contains harmful substances that can agglutinate red blood cells and interfere with the assimilation of trypsin, a digestive enzyme. Therefore, it is crucial to cook soy well to destroy these substances. Additionally, soy contains goitrogens, which can cause goiter in specific individuals, but these substances are also destroyed when cooked.

Hypertension and Fundus Hemorrhage
Tomato (Lycopersicon esculentum)

To harness the benefits of tomatoes, consume 1 or 2 fresh raw tomatoes on an empty stomach for 15 days. However, caution is advised when consuming unripe tomatoes, as they contain tomatidine, which can harm health. These green tomatoes should not be eaten. Consuming tomatoes in excess can cause nausea, vomiting, excessive salivation, and fatigue. In severe cases, excessive ingestion of unripe tomatoes can even be fatal. Note that as the tomato ripens, the tomatidine decreases or disappears altogether.

Additionally, consuming raw tomatoes on an empty stomach is not recommended, as their gelatinous substances can mix with gastric juice and cause discomfort. People with stomach or spleen weakness and diarrhea should also avoid consuming raw tomatoes. These precautions are essential to prevent any adverse reactions to tomato ingestion.

Additional Remedies

In addition to the foods already mentioned, there are other natural remedies that can complement your efforts to manage blood pressure effectively. Here are some highly effective options:

▸ **Onion and Garlic**

Adding more onions and garlic to your diet can be incredibly beneficial. These foods not only help lower blood pressure but also reduce cholesterol levels and improve blood circulation.

Practical Tip: If you're not fond of the taste of garlic or worry about bad breath, consider using odorless garlic capsules, which retain all its health benefits.

‣ Anti-Hypertension Broth

This broth is a simple, healthy, and natural way to help regulate blood pressure. The recipe includes ingredients known for their beneficial effects: one large clove of garlic, one onion, 120 grams of celery, 30 grams of chives, and 240 grams of carrots. If you have diabetes or elevated blood sugar levels, it's recommended to exclude the carrots.

Preparation: Cook all the ingredients in water without adding salt. This broth can be consumed three times a week as your sole evening meal. It not only helps lower blood pressure but also supports light and healthy eating at night.

‣ Adopt a Balanced Diet

If high blood pressure is linked to unhealthy eating habits, adopting a well-balanced diet is essential. Following the nutritional recommendations in this guide will help normalize blood pressure by consistently incorporating wholesome, nutrient-rich foods into your daily meals.

‣ Juice Fasting

A controlled fasting plan based on natural juices over several days can also be highly effective in detoxifying the body, regulating blood pressure, and enhancing overall health and well-being.

By incorporating these additional remedies alongside a balanced diet and the hypertension-friendly foods mentioned earlier, you can establish a holistic approach to naturally improving your vascular health and promoting overall wellness.

Caffeine and Hypertension: Ally or Silent Enemy?

The relationship between caffeine consumption and hypertension has long been a subject of controversy, both within the scientific community and among the general public. Found in coffee, tea, soft drinks, and energy drinks, caffeine is a powerful central nervous system stimulant and a daily ritual for millions of people. However, its impact on cardiovascular health–especially blood pressure–has raised questions and fueled ongoing debate.

While some research indicates that caffeine can cause a temporary increase in blood pressure, particularly in sensitive individuals, other studies emphasize its antioxidant and neuroprotective benefits when consumed in moderation. This section provides an in-depth exploration of the advantages and disadvantages of caffeine in relation to hypertension, based on current scientific evidence and expert opinions in the healthcare industry.

‣ The mechanism of action of caffeine:

Caffeine primarily antagonistically affects adenosine receptors in the brain. Adenosine is a neurotransmitter that promotes sleep and relaxation by inhibiting neuronal activity. By blocking these receptors, caffeine releases neurotransmitters, such as dopamine and norepinephrine, which are responsible for its stimulant effects.

In terms of its cardiovascular impact, caffeine can cause a temporary increase in blood pressure. This is due in part to its ability to increase the release of catecholamines, such as adrenaline, which in turn can increase heart rate and peripheral vascular resistance, factors that contribute to increased blood pressure.

‣ Scientific evidence: Conflicting studies:

The scientific evidence on the relationship between caffeine and blood pressure is contradictory. Some studies have shown that regular caffeine consumption can lead to a moderate increase in blood pressure, while others have found no significant long-term relationship.

- **Short-term studies**: Several studies have shown that caffeine intake can increase systolic and diastolic blood pressure in the short term, generally between 3 and 15 mmHg. This effect may be more pronounced in people who do not consume caffeine regularly or are sensitive to its effects.

- **Long-term effects**: The evidence on the long-term impact of caffeine consumption on blood pressure is less clear. Some longitudinal studies suggest that regular caffeine consumption is not associated with a sustained increase in blood pressure, while others suggest that it may contribute to the develop-ment of hypertension, especially in genetically predisposed people.

- **Meta-analyses and systematic reviews**: Meta-analyses have attempted to consolidate these divergent findings. Some conclude that moderate caffeine consumption has no significant effect on the risk of hypertension, while others suggest a slightly elevated risk.

▸ Factors Influencing the Response to Caffeine:

Individual response to caffeine can vary significantly due to several factors, including genetics, age, gender, and the presence of underlying medical conditions.

- **Genetics**: Genetic variations in adenosine receptors or in the enzymes that metabolize caffeine may influence individual sensitivity to caffeine and its impact on blood pressure.

- **Habitual Consumption**: People who regularly consume caffeine may develop a tolerance to its effects on blood pressure, while non-consumers may experience a more pronounced increase.

- **Age and Gender**: Some studies suggest that women may be more sensitive to caffeine's effects on blood pressure than men and that sensitivity may decrease with age.

▸ Expert Perspectives:

The medical and scientific community has varied opinions on the relationship between caffeine and high blood pressure. While some experts emphasize the need for caution, especially in people with pre-existing hypertension, others conclude that moderate caffeine consumption can be part of a healthy diet for most people.

- **Precautions for people with hypertension**: Experts often advise limiting caffeine intake and observing any changes in blood pressure for those diagnosed with hypertension. They also recommend discussing with a physician the possibility of ambulatory blood pressure monitoring to evaluate the individual effects of caffeine.

- **Risk and benefit**: Some experts argue that the potential benefits of caffeine consumption, such as improved attention and cognitive performance, may outweigh the possible risks, provided it is consumed in moderation. However, this must be balanced with consideration of individual cardiovascular risk factors.

- **Ongoing research**: Research on caffeine and blood pressure continues to evolve. Recent studies are exploring the role of the gut microbiota in caffeine metabolism and how this might influence cardiovascular response. In addition, research on the impact of caffeine consumption in different populations, including ethnic and genetic differences, is ongoing.

▸ **Final Considerations:**

The controversy over caffeine and high blood pressure highlights the importance of a personalized approach to health management. While caffeine consumption may be harmless for some people, others may find that it significantly impacts their blood pressure.

▸ **Practical recommendations:**

- **Self-monitoring**: People concerned about caffeine's effects on their blood pressure should practice self-monitoring, recording their blood pressure levels before and after caffeine consumption to identify any significant patterns.

- **Education and awareness**: Education about the potential effects of caffeine and the importance of moderate consumption can help them make informed decisions about their diet and lifestyle.

▸ **Conclusion:**

The relationship between caffeine and high blood pressure remains a nuanced and multifaceted topic. Despite extensive research, reaching definitive answers is challenging due to varying individual responses and the numerous factors influencing cardiovascular health. However, one consistent takeaway is that moderate caffeine consumption is generally safe for most individuals when personal health conditions and lifestyle choices are taken into account. The key lies in practicing moderation and being mindful of how caffeine affects your body and overall well-being.

Ultimately, as with most areas of health and nutrition, a balanced and informed approach is essential for enjoying caffeine's benefits while minimizing potential risks. Going forward, advancing research will likely provide a more refined and personalized understanding of how to best manage caffeine consumption in relation to blood pressure and cardiovascular health.

Beneficial Foods and Beverages

If you have high blood pressure, maintaining a healthy diet is essential for keeping your blood pressure under control and safeguarding your cardiovascular health. A balanced diet, rich in specific foods and beverages, can not only help regulate blood pressure but also lower the risk of related complications. Here is a selection of options to support your overall well-being:

▸ **Fruits and vegetables**: Fruits and vegetables are essential in a diet to control blood pressure. They are rich in nutrients, fiber, and antioxidants that promote cardiovascular health. Vibrantly colored fruits and vegetables, such as berries, citrus fruits, tomatoes, spinach, and broccoli, are especially beneficial because of their vitamin C, potassium, and other heart-healthy compounds.

▸ **Whole grains**: Whole grains, such as oats, brown rice, whole wheat, and quinoa, are sources of fiber and essential nutrients that can help lower blood pressure. The soluble fiber in whole grains helps lower cholesterol, vital to maintaining a healthy cardiovascular system.

▸ **Fish rich in omega-3 fatty acids**: Fish such as salmon, trout, tuna, and sardines are rich in omega-3 fatty acids, which have anti-inflammatory properties and can help lower blood pressure. Consuming fish at least twice a week is recommended as part of a heart-healthy diet.

▸ **Low-fat dairy**: Low-fat dairy products, such as skim milk, low-fat yogurt, and low-fat cheeses, are sources of calcium and healthy protein. If you do not have specific dietary restrictions, these foods can be part of a balanced diet for blood pressure control.

▸ **Legumes**: Legumes, such as beans, lentils, and chickpeas, are excellent sources of vegetable protein, fiber, and minerals such as potassium and magnesium. These nutrients can help regulate blood pressure, control weight, and reduce the risk of cardiovascular disease.

▸ **Nuts and seeds**: Nuts and seeds, such as almonds, walnuts, chia seeds, and flax seeds, are rich in healthy fatty acids, fiber, and minerals. These foods can benefit cardiovascular health and may help lower blood pressure.

▸ **Healthy beverages**: Besides drinking enough water, some beverages may benefit people with high blood pressure. For example, Green and hibiscus tea have been associated with lowering blood pressure. Limiting the consumption of sugary drinks and opting for options without added sugar is also recommended.

Foods and Beverages to Limit or Avoid

Managing high blood pressure requires being mindful of the foods and beverages that may aggravate the condition. Cutting back on or completely removing certain items from your diet can have a meaningful impact on maintaining healthy blood pressure levels and reducing the risk of cardiovascular complications. Below is a list of items to limit or avoid:

▸ **Salt**: Excessive salt consumption is a significant contributor to high blood pressure. Salt contains sodium, which retains fluids in the body and increases blood pressure. Salty foods such as processed foods, sausages, canned foods, salty snacks, and sodium-rich condiments such as soy sauce should be reduced.

▸ **Foods high in saturated and trans fats**: These fats are found mainly in animal products, such as red meat, full-fat dairy products, butter, and commercial baked goods. Saturated and trans fats can clog arteries and increase the risk of cardiovascular disease.

▸ **Sugar and sugary foods**: Excessive consumption of sugar can increase the risk of developing high blood pressure and other heart-related diseases. Sugary foods and beverages such as soft drinks, commercial fruit juices, cakes, cookies, and candies should be limited.

▸ **Alcoholic beverages**: Excessive alcohol consumption can raise blood pressure and damage the heart. It is recommended to limit alcohol intake to moderate amounts, which is a maximum of one alcoholic drink per day for women and two alcoholic beverages per day for men.

▸ **Coffee* and caffeinated beverages**: Caffeine can temporarily increase blood pressure and make the heart beat faster. Although the effects may vary from person to person, reducing the consumption of coffee and other caffeinated beverages, such as tea or energy drinks, is recommended.

▸ **Processed foods and fast foods**: Processed foods and fast foods often contain high levels of sodium, saturated fats, and trans fats, as well as additives and preservatives. These foods are unhealthy and can contribute to the development of high blood pressure and other chronic diseases.

It is important to note that each person may have different food sensitivities and reactions.

Healthy Substitutes to Reduce Salt Intake

Cutting back on table salt doesn't mean sacrificing flavor. In fact, there are plenty of spices, herbs, and seasonings that can enhance the taste of your dishes in a healthier way. Here are some specific recommendations based on the type of food:

▸ **For meat:** Instead of using salt, opt for spices like bay leaf, nutmeg, black pepper, sage, thyme, garlic, onion, oregano, or rosemary. These herbs deliver a wide range of flavors that can elevate your dishes.

▸ **For fish:** Bring out the flavor in fish dishes with alternatives such as curry powder, dill, mustard, lemon juice, or black pepper. These ingredients provide fresh and aromatic notes without the need for salt.

▸ **For vegetables:** Add an extra layer of flavor to your vegetables by using herbs like rosemary, sage, dill, cinnamon, tarragon, basil, or parsley. These options will help you enjoy complex and vibrant flavors in your veggie dishes.

These natural, sodium-free seasonings not only enhance the variety in your meals but also help you maintain better control over your blood pressure.

Hypertension Support: Easy and Tasty Recipes

Healthy eating doesn't have to be boring. Here are some delicious, easy-to-make recipes specifically designed for those looking to manage their blood pressure. Perfect for enjoying while prioritizing your health!

Breakfast Options

1. Oatmeal with Fresh Berries and Nuts
Cook a serving of rolled oats with water or low-fat milk.
Top with fresh berries like blueberries or strawberries.
Add a small handful of unsalted nuts like almonds or walnuts for crunch.
Optional: Sprinkle with a dash of cinnamon for extra flavor.

2. Avocado Toast on Whole Grain Bread
Mash half an avocado and spread it on a slice of whole-grain bread.
Top with slices of tomato and a sprinkle of black pepper.
Optionally, add a poached or boiled egg for extra protein.

3. Smoothie Bowl
Blend one banana, a handful of spinach, and a cup of unsweetened almond milk or low-fat yogurt.
Pour into a bowl and top with sliced kiwi, chia seeds, and a small granola.

4. Greek Yogurt Parfait
Use low-fat Greek yogurt as a base.
Layer with fresh fruit like peaches, pears, or berries.
Top with a sprinkle of flaxseeds or chia seeds.

5. Veggie Omelette
Whisk together egg whites or a combination of whole eggs and egg whites.
Pour into a non-stick pan and add chopped vegetables like spinach, bell peppers, and onions.
Cook until set and fold over. Serve with a slice of whole-grain toast.

6. Quinoa Breakfast Bowl
Cook quinoa according to package instructions.
Mix with a splash of almond milk, a handful of chopped nuts, and fresh apple slices.
Sprinkle with cinnamon and a few raisins for sweetness.

7. Whole Grain Pancakes with Berries
Prepare whole-grain pancake batter from scratch or use a low-sodium mix.
Serve with a topping of fresh berries and a drizzle of pure maple syrup or honey.

8. Chia Seed Pudding
Mix chia seeds with almond milk and sit in the refrigerator overnight.
In the morning, top with sliced banana and a sprinkle of cinnamon.

9. Spinach and Mushroom Frittata
Sauté spinach and sliced mushrooms in a non-stick pan with olive oil.
Beat eggs or egg whites with a splash of milk and pour over the

vegetables.
Cook on low heat until set, then finish under a broiler for a few minutes.

10. Banana and Almond Butter Toast
Spread a thin layer of unsweetened almond butter on whole-grain bread.
Top with banana slices and a sprinkle of flaxseeds or chia seeds.

11. Cottage Cheese with Pineapple and Walnuts
Use low-fat cottage cheese as a base.
Add chunks of fresh or canned pineapple (in juice, not syrup).
Top with a few walnuts for added texture and omega-3.

12. Buckwheat Pancakes with Apple Compote
Make pancakes using buckwheat flour.
For the compote, cook chopped apples with water and cinnamon until soft.
Serve the pancakes topped with the apple compote.

13. Berry and Spinach Smoothie
Blend a cup of mixed berries, a handful of spinach, half a banana, and almond milk or water.
Optionally, add a tablespoon of flaxseeds or chia seeds for extra nutrition.

14. Whole Grain English Muffin with Tomato and Basil
Toast a whole-grain English muffin.
Top with slices of fresh tomato, a few fresh basil leaves, and a drizzle of olive oil.

15. Muesli with Almond Milk
Combine rolled oats, dried fruits (like raisins or dried apricots), nuts, and seeds.
Serve with unsweetened almond milk and fresh fruit toppings.

16. Quinoa and Fruit Salad
Cook quinoa and let it cool.
Mix with various fresh fruits such as oranges, grapes, and berries.
Add a squeeze of lemon or lime juice for extra flavor.

Lunch Creations

1. Grilled Chicken Salad
Grill a skinless chicken breast and slice it thinly.
Serve over mixed greens with cherry tomatoes, cucumbers, and bell peppers.
Dress with a homemade vinaigrette of olive oil, lemon juice, and herbs.

2. Quinoa and Black Bean Bowl
Cook quinoa and mix with black beans, corn, diced red onion, and chopped cilantro.
Dress with lime juice and a little olive oil.
Optionally, add diced avocado for creaminess.

3. Lentil Soup
In low-sodium vegetable broth, cook lentils with chopped carrots, celery, tomatoes, and spinach.
Season with garlic, cumin, and a bay leaf for flavor.
Serve with a slice of whole-grain bread.

4. Turkey and Avocado Wrap
Fill a whole-grain tortilla with sliced turkey breast, avocado, lettuce, and tomato.
Roll up tightly and serve with a side of carrot sticks or a small salad.

5. Vegetable Stir-Fry with Tofu
Sauté tofu cubes and a mix of your favorite vegetables (like broccoli, bell peppers, and snap peas) in a bit of olive oil.
Season with low-sodium soy sauce and a sprinkle of sesame seeds.
Serve over brown rice or quinoa.

6. Chickpea Salad Sandwich
Mash-cooked chickpeas and mix with diced celery, red onion, a little mustard, and lemon juice.
Serve on whole grain bread with lettuce and tomato slices.

7. Mediterranean Couscous Salad
Cook whole wheat couscous and mix with cherry tomatoes, cucumber, red onion, olives, and feta cheese.
Dress with olive oil, lemon juice, and fresh herbs like parsley or mint.

8. Stuffed Bell Peppers
Halve and hollow out bell peppers.
Fill with brown rice, black beans, diced tomatoes, and spices.
Bake until the peppers are tender.

9. Spinach and Feta Stuffed Chicken Breast
Stuff a chicken breast with spinach, feta cheese, and herbs.
Bake until the chicken is cooked through.
Serve with a side of roasted vegetables.

10. Zucchini Noodles with Pesto
Spiralize zucchini into noodles.
Toss with homemade or store-bought low-sodium pesto.
Optionally, top with cherry tomatoes and pine nuts.

11. Baked Sweet Potato with Black Beans
Bake a sweet potato until tender.
Top with black beans, diced tomatoes, avocado, and a sprinkle of cilantro.
Add a squeeze of lime for extra flavor.

12. Eggplant and Chickpea Stew
Sauté eggplant cubes with onion, garlic, and tomatoes.
Add canned chickpeas (rinsed) and spices like cumin and paprika.
Simmer until the eggplant is soft and serve with whole grain bread.

13. Whole Wheat Pasta Primavera
Cook whole wheat pasta and toss with sautéed vegetables such as zucchini, bell peppers, and spinach.
Add a drizzle of olive oil and a sprinkle of Parmesan cheese.

14. Cauliflower Rice Bowl
Sauté riced cauliflower with garlic and a mix of vegetables like bell peppers, peas, and carrots.
Top with a poached egg and a sprinkle of sesame seeds.

15. Salmon and Avocado Salad
Grill or bake salmon fillets.
Serve over a bed of mixed greens with avocado slices, cucumber, and a squeeze of lemon juice.

16. Falafel Wrap
Use whole grain pita or wrap and fill with baked falafel, lettuce, tomatoes, and cucumber.
Add a dollop of low-fat yogurt or tzatziki sauce.

17. Vegetable and Hummus Plate
Serve a variety of fresh vegetables, such as carrots, bell peppers, and cherry tomatoes, with a side of hummus.

Add whole-grain pita bread for dipping.

18. Spinach and Mushroom Quesadilla
Fill a whole grain tortilla with sautéed spinach, mushrooms, and a small amount of cheese.

Grill until the tortilla is crispy and the cheese is melted. Serve with salsa.

19. Beet and Orange Salad
Combine cooked beets with orange slices and arugula. Dress with olive oil and balsamic vinegar.

20. Broccoli and Cheese Soup
Make a soup using low-sodium broth, broccoli, and a small amount of low-fat cheese.

Puree for a creamy texture and serve with whole-grain crackers.

21. Roasted Vegetable and Couscous Salad
Roast a mix of vegetables such as zucchini, red bell peppers, and carrots.

Toss with whole wheat couscous and dress with lemon juice, olive oil, and fresh herbs.

22. Chicken and Vegetable Stir-Fry
Stir-fry slices of chicken breast with broccoli, bell peppers, and snow peas in a bit of olive oil.

Add a splash of low-sodium soy sauce and serve over brown rice.

23. Tomato and Cucumber Gazpacho
Blend fresh tomatoes, cucumber, red bell pepper, onion, garlic, and a splash of vinegar.

Chill and serve cold, garnished with fresh herbs like basil or parsley.

24. Egg Salad Lettuce Wraps
Make egg salad with chopped boiled eggs, a little mustard, and Greek yogurt.

Serve in large lettuce leaves instead of bread.

25. Mushroom and Barley Risotto
Cook pearl barley with mushrooms, onions, and garlic in low-sodium vegetable broth.

Stir until creamy and finish with a sprinkle of fresh herbs.

26. Turkey and Spinach Stuffed Bell Peppers
Stuff bell peppers with ground turkey, spinach, diced tomatoes, and herbs.
Bake until the peppers are tender and the filling is cooked through.

27. Avocado and White Bean Wrap
Mash avocado and mix with white beans, diced red onion, and a squeeze of lime juice.
Spread on a whole grain wrap and top with spinach leaves.

28. Roasted Red Pepper and Lentil Soup
Simmer red lentils with roasted red peppers, tomatoes, and spices like cumin and coriander.
Blend until smooth and serve with a side of whole-grain bread.

29. Spring Roll Salad
Combine shredded carrots, cucumber, bell peppers, and rice noodles.
Dress with a light vinaigrette of lime juice, fish sauce (low-sodium), and a bit of honey.
Top with fresh mint and cilantro.

30. Eggplant and Tomato Pita Pizza
Top whole-grain pita bread with sliced eggplant, tomato sauce, and a sprinkle of low-fat mozzarella.
Bake until the cheese is melted and bubbly.

These lunch ideas focus on incorporating plenty of vegetables, lean proteins, and whole grains while keeping sodium levels low to support healthy blood pressure management.

Snacks

1. Grilled Chicken Salad
Grill a skinless chicken breast and slice it thinly.
Serve over mixed greens with cherry tomatoes, cucumbers, and bell peppers.
Dress with a homemade vinaigrette of olive oil, lemon juice, and herbs.

2. Quinoa and Black Bean Bowl

Cook quinoa and mix with black beans, corn, diced red onion, and chopped cilantro.
Dress with lime juice and a little olive oil.
Optionally, add diced avocado for creaminess.

3. Lentil Soup
In low-sodium vegetable broth, cook lentils with chopped carrots, celery, tomatoes, and spinach.
Season with garlic, cumin, and a bay leaf for flavor.
Serve with a slice of whole-grain bread.

4. Turkey and Avocado Wrap
Fill a whole-grain tortilla with sliced turkey breast, avocado, lettuce, and tomato.
Roll up tightly and serve with a side of carrot sticks or a small salad.

5. Vegetable Stir-Fry with Tofu
Sauté tofu cubes and a mix of your favorite vegetables (like broccoli, bell peppers, and snap peas) in a bit of olive oil.
Season with low-sodium soy sauce and a sprinkle of sesame seeds.
Serve over brown rice or quinoa.

6. Chickpea Salad Sandwich
Mash-cooked chickpeas and mix with diced celery, red onion, a little mustard, and lemon juice.
Serve on whole grain bread with lettuce and tomato slices.

7. Mediterranean Couscous Salad
Cook whole wheat couscous and mix with cherry tomatoes, cucumber, red onion, olives, and feta cheese.
Dress with olive oil, lemon juice, and fresh herbs like parsley or mint.

8. Stuffed Bell Peppers
Halve and hollow out bell peppers.
Fill with brown rice, black beans, diced tomatoes, and spices.
Bake until the peppers are tender.

9. Spinach and Feta Stuffed Chicken Breast
Stuff a chicken breast with spinach, feta cheese, and herbs.
Bake until the chicken is cooked through.
Serve with a side of roasted vegetables.

10. Zucchini Noodles with Pesto
Spiralize zucchini into noodles.

Toss with homemade or store-bought low-sodium pesto.
Optionally, top with cherry tomatoes and pine nuts.

Dinner Ideas

1. Baked Chicken with Spinach and Tomatoes
Season chicken breasts with garlic, basil, and oregano.
Top with fresh spinach leaves and diced tomatoes.
Bake until the chicken is cooked, and serve with a side of quinoa.

2. Zucchini Noodles with Avocado Sauce
Spiralize zucchini into noodles.
Blend ripe avocado with lime juice, garlic, and cilantro for a creamy sauce.
Toss the zucchini noodles with the avocado sauce and top with cherry tomatoes.

3. Roasted Vegetable and Quinoa Bowl
Roast a mix of non-starchy vegetables like bell peppers, broccoli, and cauliflower.
Serve over a bed of quinoa and drizzle with a lemon-tahini dressing.

4. Grilled Salmon with Asparagus
Season salmon fillets with dill, lemon juice, and pepper.
Grill alongside asparagus spears until the salmon is cooked through.
Serve with a small side of brown rice.

5. Eggplant and Lentil Stew
Simmer eggplant cubes with lentils, diced tomatoes, and spices like cumin and coriander in vegetable broth.
Serve hot with a sprinkle of fresh parsley.

6. Turkey and Vegetable Stir-Fry
Stir-fry lean ground turkey with various non-starchy vegetables such as bok choy, bell peppers, and mushrooms.
Season with ginger and low-sodium soy sauce.
Serve over a small portion of brown rice or quinoa.

7. Stuffed Bell Peppers with Cauliflower Rice
Hollow out bell peppers with cauliflower rice, black beans, and

diced tomatoes.
Bake until the peppers are tender.

8. Lemon Herb Cod with Broccoli
Bake cod fillets with lemon slices and fresh herbs like thyme and rosemary.
Serve with steamed broccoli and a small serving of whole-grain pasta.

9. Chickpea and Spinach Curry
Cook chickpeas with spinach, tomatoes, and curry spices in coconut milk.
Serve over a portion of brown rice or quinoa.

10. Tofu and Vegetable Skewers
Marinate tofu cubes and vegetables like zucchini and cherry tomatoes in olive oil and herbs.
Grill until the tofu is golden and the vegetables are tender, and serve with a side of wild rice.

11. Grilled Chicken and Vegetable Salad
Grill chicken breast and vegetables like zucchini, bell peppers, and red onions.
Slice and serve over a bed of mixed greens with a balsamic vinaigrette.

12. Baked Trout with Almonds
Season trout fillets with lemon juice, garlic, and chopped almonds.
Bake until the fish is cooked, and serve with steamed green beans and a small serving of wild rice.

13. Cauliflower and Mushroom Stir-Fry
Stir-fry cauliflower florets and sliced mushrooms with garlic and ginger.
Add a splash of low-sodium soy sauce and serve over a small portion of brown rice.

14. Turkey Lettuce Wraps
Sauté ground turkey with water chestnuts, green onions, and ginger.
Serve in large lettuce leaves with a drizzle of hoisin sauce.

15. Vegetable and Chickpea Soup
Simmer chickpeas with carrots, celery, and kale in a low-sodium vegetable broth.
Season with herbs like thyme and rosemary and serve hot.

16. Spinach and Feta Stuffed Chicken
Stuff chicken breasts with spinach and feta cheese.
Bake until the chicken is cooked, and serve with roasted Brussels sprouts.

17. Shrimp and Avocado Salad
Grill shrimp seasoned with lime and chili powder.
Serve over a salad of avocado, mixed greens, and cherry tomatoes with a lime vinaigrette.

18. Sweet Potato and Black Bean Tacos
Roast sweet potato cubes and mix with black beans.
Serve in corn tortillas with sliced avocado and fresh cilantro.

19. Broccoli and Cashew Stir-Fry
Stir-fry broccoli and bell peppers with cashews in sesame oil.
Season with low-sodium soy sauce and serve over a small portion of quinoa.

20. Basil Pesto Zoodles with Cherry Tomatoes
Spiralize zucchini into noodles.
Toss with homemade basil pesto and halved cherry tomatoes.

21. Herb-Roasted Chicken Thighs with Brussels Sprouts
Season chicken thighs with rosemary, thyme, and garlic.
Roast alongside halved Brussels sprouts until the chicken is cooked and the sprouts are caramelized.

22. Mushroom and Spinach Frittata
Sauté mushrooms and spinach, then add beaten eggs.
Cook until set and serve with a side of mixed greens.

23. Grilled Eggplant with Tomato and Feta
Grill slices of eggplant and top with diced tomatoes, crumbled feta, and fresh basil.
Drizzle with balsamic reduction before serving.

24. Lentil and Vegetable Shepherd's Pie
Cook lentils with carrots, peas, and onions in vegetable broth.
Top with a layer of mashed cauliflower and bake until golden.

25. Roasted Red Pepper and Tomato Soup
Blend roasted red peppers and tomatoes with garlic and herbs.
Simmer and serve hot, garnished with fresh basil.

26. Chicken and Vegetable Kabobs
Skewer chunks of chicken breast with bell peppers, onions, and

cherry tomatoes.

Grill until the chicken is cooked, and serve with a side of quinoa.

27. Tofu and Broccoli Curry

Cook tofu cubes and broccoli florets in curry spices and coconut milk.

Serve over a small portion of brown rice or cauliflower rice.

28. Grilled Portobello Mushroom Burgers

Marinate Portobello mushrooms in balsamic vinegar and grill.
Serve on whole grain buns with lettuce, tomato, and avocado.

29. Zucchini and Tomato Gratin

Layer slices of zucchini and tomato in a baking dish.
Top with a sprinkle of Parmesan cheese and bake until tender.

30. Curried Cauliflower and Pea Salad

Roast cauliflower florets with curry powder.

Toss with green peas, fresh cilantro, and a light yogurt dressing.

JUICES & SMOOTHIES

"Optimal nutrition is the medicine of tomorrow" (Dr. Linus Pauling)

Raw foods, often referred to as "living" foods, are an exceptional source of vitamins, minerals, fiber, trace elements, enzymes, and other vital compounds that support overall health. Incorporating these nutrient-rich foods into your daily diet not only aids in disease prevention but also alleviates symptoms of various health conditions, slows down the aging process, balances gut flora, and enhances energy levels and vitality.

While salads, whole fruits, and nuts are excellent raw food options, one of the easiest and most convenient ways to ensure regular intake is by preparing homemade juices, smoothies, and shakes. These beverages serve as a delicious and practical alternative for individuals who may not enjoy consuming fruits and vegetables directly, making it easier to include these essential nutrients in their diet.

In today's world, where ultra-processed foods and toxins have become increasingly prevalent, the need for natural, nutrient-dense foods is more crucial than ever. Raw foods play a vital role in supporting detoxification, maintaining health, and restoring balance to the body.

Many people tend to prepare their juices and smoothies using only fruits, often overlooking the incredible health benefits vegetables and leafy greens provide. Adding these to your recipes not only increases variety but also significantly boosts their nutritional value, enhancing their antioxidant, remineralizing, toning, and alkalizing properties. These qualities help maintain the body's balance, rejuvenate cells, and promote overall well-being. Additionally, vegetables and greens lower the glycemic index, improve satiety, and maximize the health benefits of these preparations.

However, it is crucial to understand that most store-bought juices are far from healthy options. These commercial products are often loaded with excessive added sugars, artificial sweeteners, preservatives, and harmful chemical additives. Furthermore, the pasteurization processes used during production strip away essential vitamins and enzymes, rendering them nutritionally deficient. The high level of refinement also removes fiber, a vital component of whole foods. In many cases, these juices contain only minimal amounts of actual fruit, making them highly processed and lacking true nutritional value.

One major concern with many juices and smoothies is their high glycemic index, which can cause blood sugar spikes, lead to weight gain, and contribute to long-term metabolic imbalances. To truly enjoy healthy and nourishing beverages, the best approach is to prepare them at home using fresh, natural, and high-quality ingredients. Homemade juices and smoothies are packed with nutrients that provide genuine benefits for your body and overall well-being.

Incorporating fresh juices made from fruits, vegetables, and leafy greens into your daily routine is an excellent practice for maintaining a healthy and energetic body. With endless combinations to explore, you can enjoy not only flavorful and refreshing options but also targeted health benefits, such as relief from conditions like arthritis, thanks to essential nutrients that support wellness. Making this a part of your everyday life can transform your health, boost your energy, and elevate your quality of life. Try it for yourself and feel the difference!

Juices: Unleash Their Power

Incorporating smoothies or shakes into your diet can be a fantastic way to boost your health. Below are some of their most significant benefits:

▸ **Compliance with Recommended Fruit and Vegetable Intake**: Smoothies and shakes offer a practical and enjoyable way to meet the daily recommendation of five servings of fruits and vegetables. They provide a diverse range of essential nutrients that support optimal health and overall well-being.

▸ **Easy Assimilation and Digestion**: As liquid meals, smoothies and shakes are gentler on the digestive system and allow for quicker nutrient absorption. They are especially beneficial for individuals with digestive sensitivities or challenges.

- **Vitamin and Mineral Powerhouse**: Made from fresh fruits and vegetables, smoothies and shakes are rich sources of essential vitamins and minerals that promote the proper functioning of the body.

- **Detoxification and Cleansing**: Ingredients like leafy greens and natural antioxidants help flush out toxins, enhance cell health, and support effective internal cleansing.

- **Balancing Body pH**: By incorporating alkaline foods, smoothies and shakes play a key role in stabilizing the body's pH levels, aiding disease prevention and improving overall wellness.

- **Reduction of Inflammation**: Anti-inflammatory additions such as turmeric, ginger, and leafy greens can help minimize inflammation, fostering better health and increased comfort.

- **A Balanced Meal Replacement**: When combined with protein, healthy fats, and complex carbohydrates, smoothies become a nourishing and balanced meal replacement. They provide sustained energy and promote fullness throughout the day.

- **Supports Weight Management**: With their low-calorie yet nutrient-dense profiles, smoothies and shakes encourage healthy eating habits. They help manage appetite and support maintaining or achieving an ideal weight.

- **Enhances Skin Health**: Packed with skin-friendly vitamins like A and C from fresh ingredients, smoothies and shakes contribute to hydrated, radiant, and healthy skin.

- **Slows Cellular Aging**: The antioxidants in smoothie ingredients combat oxidative damage, protect cells, and help maintain a youthful appearance.

- **Boosts Energy and Vitality**: Smoothies made with superfoods provide a steady energy boost, helping you stay active, energized, and revitalized throughout the day.

In conclusion, smoothies and shakes are a nutritious, convenient, and versatile addition to your diet. Not only do they make it easier to meet your daily fruit and vegetable intake, but they also offer a wide array of health benefits. Packed with essential nutrients, they support overall well-being–all while being refreshing, delicious, and easy to enjoy.

Homemade vs. Commercial Juices

Nowadays, identifying which foods truly benefit our health can be quite challenging. Supermarkets are overflowing with an extensive range of options, flaunting attractive packaging and clever designs that promise to be natural and healthy. While advertising and packaging often catch our attention, are we genuinely purchasing natural beverages made from fruits and vegetables? Do you know the key differences between homemade juices and industrial products? Are packaged products really as nutritious as they claim to be? Taking a few moments to carefully read ingredient labels and analyze their composition may uncover some surprising truths.

A few years ago, international regulations were established to define the standards that every fruit-based beverage must meet, specifying precise characteristics for each type of product. Below, we'll explore these distinctions and delve into the essential differences.

‣ Fruit Juice

Fruit juice is derived from fresh, chilled, or frozen fruits without undergoing any fermentation. It may contain separately extracted pulp and, in some cases, be blended with juice from various fruits. Labels are required to specify the composition in descending order, including the exact percentage of each fruit.

To prolong shelf life and eliminate the need for refrigeration, fruit juice is typically sterilized or pasteurized. Unfortunately, these processes result in significant nutrient loss, particularly impacting essential vitamins and enzymes. Moreover, the juice lacks the natural fiber found in whole fruits.

‣ Juice from Concentrates

Juice from concentrates is created by reconstituting dehydrated juice concentrates with water. Concentrates are produced by extracting natural juice through evaporation or other physical methods. During reconstitution, manufacturers may add aromas or pulp from similar fruits to partially restore flavor.

Though widely consumed, these juices suffer nutrient losses during production, including enzymes, vitamins, minerals, and the valuable fiber that characterizes natural fruit.

‣ Dehydrated or Powdered Fruit Juice

This product is manufactured by removing water from fruit to create a dry powder, which can later be rehydrated or sold in its dehydrated state. However, the dehydration process significantly diminishes its nutritional value, leading to the loss of enzymes, vitamins, minerals, and natural fiber.

‣ Fruit Nectar
Fruit nectar differs from pure juice as it is made using fruit concentrate, water, and added sugars or sweeteners. Its nutritional value is considerably lower compared to natural fruit juices due to its inclusion of artificial additives to enhance flavor, color, or shelf life.

‣ Juice-Based Drinks
These beverages typically combine various fruits but contain minimal actual fruit juice. Often, they lack the essential nutrients derived from fruits, consisting largely of water, artificial aromas, colorings, and sweeteners.

‣ Milk-Infused Juice Drinks
Milk-infused juice drinks include fruit juice, often from concentrates, in very small proportions. They are mixed with milk, water, flavorings, and other ingredients. These beverages are not considered true juices, and any nutrients present are artificially added during manufacturing to compensate for losses incurred during processing.

‣ Vegetable and/or Greens Juice
Vegetable and greens juices are extracted from vegetables using specialized industrial methods, often with added pulp or pureed ingredients. They may also blend various vegetables to create balanced or palatable flavors.

To extend shelf life and eliminate refrigeration requirements, these juices undergo pasteurization or sterilization, which unfortunately reduces essential nutrients, including vitamins and phytonutrients. Additionally, they lack the natural fiber of whole vegetables and may include preservatives, salt, or flavor enhancers that compromise their nutritional profile.

‣ Commercial Smoothies
Commercial smoothies are typically prepared by blending fruits, vegetables, and greens—often using purees or concentrates—with water, milk, plant-based beverages, or similar liquids. Their thicker texture comes from a higher proportion of pulp or fiber-rich components.

To enhance taste, appearance, and shelf life, industrial smoothies usually contain added sugars, preservatives, colorings, and flavorings that alter their natural composition. Moreover, they undergo pasteurization or thermal sterilization to allow room-temperature storage, further degrading their original nutrients and reducing their overall nutritional quality.

Advantages of Homemade Juices

After discovering what commercial products truly contain, it becomes evident that making juices at home offers numerous advantages. Here are the key benefits:

▸ **Complete Control Over Ingredients**: Preparing your own juices allows you to ensure the quality of the ingredients you use. There are no unnecessary additives, no preservatives, and –most importantly–no unpleasant surprises.

▸ **Variety and Creativity**: You have the freedom to choose your favorite fruits and vegetables, experiment with unique combinations, or incorporate fresh, seasonal produce. This not only provides a burst of delicious flavors but also boosts your intake of essential nutrients.

▸ **Authentic Aroma and Flavor**: Homemade juices retain the genuine aroma and taste of fresh fruits and vegetables. There's truly nothing like enjoying a freshly made juice packed with natural freshness.

▸ **Maximum Nutrient Retention**: Vitamins, minerals, enzymes, antioxidants, and other nutrients remain intact when you prepare juices at home, significantly enhancing their health benefits.

▸ **Premium Quality Ingredients**: Choosing fresh, seasonal produce at its peak ripeness ensures optimal flavor and exceptional nutritional value.

▸ **Seasonal Food Benefits**: Consuming fruits and vegetables that are in season supports sustainability, is more cost-effective, and often results in better taste and nutritional quality.

▸ **Total Customization**: Whether using a juicer or blender, you can adjust the consistency of your juice to your liking– whether you prefer a light, clear juice or a thicker, fiber-rich option.

▸ **Kid-Friendly Option**: Homemade juices are an excellent way to incorporate fruits and vegetables into children's diets, especially for picky eaters. With creative flavors and fun presentations, you can make juices irresistible for kids.

Making juices at home provides several compelling advantages: complete control over ingredients, enhanced nutrient retention, and the flexibility to tailor your drinks to your preferences. It's also a simple yet effective way to promote healthy eating for the whole family.

Possible Adverse Effects

If you suffer from **gastritis, colitis, SIBO, irritable bowel syndrome, or constipation**, it's essential to take certain precautions when preparing smoothies or juices. Following these recommendations will help you enjoy their benefits without worsening your symptoms:

▸ **Use a juicer instead of a blender**: For digestive health conditions, it's often better to use a juicer rather than a blender when making juices. Juicing removes most of the fiber from the ingredients, resulting in a smoother liquid that is gentler on your digestive system.

▸ **Moderate your fiber intake**: Although fiber is highly beneficial for overall health, excessive consumption can lead to gas, bloating, or constipation–especially for individuals with sensitive digestion. Be mindful of the fiber content in your smoothies by limiting ingredients like fruit pulp, seeds, and whole grains.

▸ **Introduce juices gradually**: If you're unsure how your body will react, start with small portions. This enables you to monitor their effects on your digestion and adjust the recipes to suit your specific needs.

▸ **Consume juices on an empty stomach**: Drinking juices on an empty stomach can maximize nutrient absorption and aid digestion. This approach minimizes the risk of digestive discomfort and helps you fully benefit from the juice's nutrients.

▸ **Tailor recipes to your personal needs**: Everyone's digestive system is unique, and responses to certain foods can vary greatly. Pay close attention to how your body reacts after consuming juices, and adapt ingredient combinations to best support your health and well-being.

When to Take Them

There are several effective ways to incorporate juices into your routine, depending on your goals and daily habits. Below are three recommended methods:

▸ **In the morning, on an empty stomach**: Begin your day with a carefully chosen juice recipe, consuming it before eating anything else. Drinking juice on an empty stomach enhances nutrient absorption and stimulates your digestive system, helping prepare it for the rest of the day.

▸ **On an empty stomach, before meals**: Enjoy a juice approximately 30 minutes before your main meals to maximize its benefits. This practice supports digestion and boosts nutrient absorption, promoting overall health and well-being.

▸ **Juice-based fasting**: Engage in a multi-day fast consisting exclusively of juices to achieve specific health objectives or to detoxify your body. Choose 2 to 3 recipes and consume them consistently throughout the day to stay nourished and energized.

Preparation Tips

Preparing fresh juices is an easy and nutritious way to make the most of the vitamins and minerals found in fruits and vegetables. To optimize the process and ensure safety, consider the following recommendations:

▸ **Choose organic ingredients**: Whenever possible, opt for organic fruits and vegetables. They provide cleaner, pesticide-free consumption and promote a healthier lifestyle.

▸ **Wash ingredients thoroughly**: Rinse all produce carefully to remove dirt, bacteria, and chemical residues. Trim any bruised, moldy, or damaged areas to prevent contamination.

▸ **Cut ingredients into smaller pieces**: Make blending easier by chopping fruits and vegetables into smaller, manageable chunks. This helps achieve a smoother texture and shortens preparation time.

▸ **Balance ingredients with low water content**: Fruits and vegetables with low water content, such as bananas and avocados, may require pre-mixing. Start with juicier ingredients to create a liquid base, then gradually add denser items for a cohesive blend.

▸ **Peel certain fruits appropriately**: Remove citrus rinds (like those from oranges and grapefruits), as their outer layers may contain toxins. However, keep the nutrient-rich white inner layer. Peel tropical fruits, such as papayas and kiwis, especially if they are grown in regions with less stringent chemical regulations.

▸ **Discard harmful seeds**: Remove seeds from apples, as they contain trace amounts of cyanide and are unsafe to consume. On the other hand, seeds from grapes, melons, lemons, and limes are safe and offer additional health benefits.

▸ **Incorporate stems and leaves mindfully**: Many stems and leaves are nutritious, but be cautious. Avoid toxic ones, such as carrot and rhubarb leaves, which can be harmful.

▸ **Drink your juice immediately**: Freshly prepared juice is best consumed right away to minimize nutrient loss and avoid oxidation. This ensures maximum freshness and health benefits.

▸ **Remove bitter celery leaves**: Bitter celery leaves can affect the flavor of your juice. Remove them before blending the stalks to create a more balanced and enjoyable taste.

Key Recommendations

Smoothies and shakes are an excellent, healthy alternative, but to get the most out of them, it's essential to keep certain aspects in mind. Below are some key recommendations:

▸ **Moderate fruit consumption**: Fruits are a fantastic source of nutrients but also contain fructose, a natural sugar that, when consumed excessively, can impact your health. Strive for balance by moderating your fruit intake throughout the day. Additionally, avoid eating fruits at night, as the body may metabolize them less efficiently during this time.

▸ **Choose seasonal fruits**: Seasonal fruits are often more nutrient-rich, flavorful, and cost-effective. By opting for fruits in season, you can enjoy their peak freshness and nutritional benefits while saving money.

▸ **Pick compatible combinations**: Not all fruits or ingredients blend well together. Research suitable pairings to create a smoothie or shake with balanced flavors and optimal nutritional value.

‣ **Use a moderate amount of ingredients**: The simplest smoothies are often the best. Avoid overloading them with excessive ingredients, which can lead to heavy textures or digestive discomfort. Stick to recommended recipes and be mindful of proportions.

‣ **Include leafy greens and vegetables**: Incorporate leafy greens, like spinach or kale, or vegetables, such as cucumber, to lower the glycemic index and boost your drink's nutrient profile. These additions make your smoothie both healthier and more satisfying.

‣ **Use natural sweeteners in moderation**: Enjoy the natural flavors of the ingredients, but if sweetening is necessary, choose options like raw honey or pure stevia. Use them sparingly to maintain a balanced nutritional profile.

‣ **Chew your drink**: Even liquid smoothies benefit from being "chewed." This simple habit stimulates the release of digestive enzymes, helping improve nutrient absorption and reducing discomfort like bloating or indigestion.

‣ **Store properly**: For the best results, consume smoothies or shakes fresh. If storing is needed, place them in a dark, airtight container in the refrigerator, or freeze individual portions for later use.

‣ **Make them fun and personalized**: Add an enjoyable twist by freezing smoothies in molds with fun shapes–an excellent way to turn a healthy drink into a delightful treat, especially for children.

These recommendations will help you make the most of your smoothies and shakes. While the recipes provided in this book are crafted to facilitate nutrient absorption, always remember that individual needs vary. Feel free to experiment with different combinations, tailor recipes to suit your tastes, and prioritize your health and well-being. Enjoy the journey to a healthier lifestyle!

Nutritious Juice Recipes for Hypertension

▸ **Orange Juice:**
Ingredients: 2 or 3 oranges.
Preparation: Peel the oranges without removing the white pith. Cut them into pieces or segments and blend.

▸ **Orange, Strawberry, and Banana Juice:**
Ingredients: 3 oranges, 3 strawberries, 1 banana.
Preparation: Squeeze and reserve the orange juice. Wash the strawberries well and remove the leaves. Peel the banana, remove the strands, and cut into slices. Blend all the ingredients.

▸ **Melon and Banana Smoothie:**
Ingredients: 1 slice of melon and 1 banana.
Preparation: Add the melon to a blender along with the diced banana. Blend until a smooth consistency is obtained.

▸ **Watermelon Juice:**
Ingredients: 300 grams of watermelon.
Preparation: Wash the watermelon, cut it into strips, and blend, including the rind.

▸ **Blackberry and Banana Smoothie:**
Ingredients: 1 ripe banana, ½ kg of blackberries, 50 grams of tofu, and 1 tablespoon of brewer's yeast.
Preparation: Blend the blackberries. Pour the juice into a blender with the banana, tofu, and yeast. Blend until smooth. Garnish with a few blackberries, and drink one hour before bedtime.

▸ **Beet and Carrot Juice:**
Ingredients: 1 beet and 2 carrots.
Preparation: Blend the beet and carrots and drink them freshly made.

▸ **Kiwi, Lemon, Grape, and Celery Juice:**
Ingredients: 1 kiwi, 1/2 lemon, 100 grams of grapes, and 2 celery stalks.
Preparation: Peel and chop the kiwi. Peel the lemon, removing the white pith, cut into quarters, and remove the seeds. Chop the celery. Blend all the ingredients.

▸ **Cucumber and Lemon Juice:**
Ingredients: Half a cucumber and 1 lemon.
Preparation: Peel the cucumber, blend it, and add the lemon juice.

▸ Carrot, Cabbage, Parsley, and Apple Juice:
Ingredients: 4 carrots, 3 collard greens, 1 handful of parsley, and ½ seedless apple.
Preparation: Chop the parsley and cabbage and blend them with the apple and carrots.

▸ Parsley, Carrot, and Celery Juice:
Ingredients: 1 bunch of parsley, 4 carrots, and 2 celery stalks.
Preparation: Chop the parsley and blend it along with the carrots and celery.

▸ Lemon and Parsley Juice:
Ingredients: 1 whole lemon (peel included) and a bunch of parsley.
Preparation: Blend the ingredients and drink on an empty stomach.

▸ Strawberry Smoothie with Tofu:
Ingredients: ½ kg of strawberries and 200 grams of tofu.
Preparation: Blend the strawberries and then add the tofu. Blend until smooth. Garnish with a strawberry.

▸ Garlic, Parsley, Carrot, and Celery Juice:
Ingredients: 1 clove of garlic, 1 handful of parsley, 4 carrots, 2 celery stalks, and 1 parsley leaf for garnish.
Preparation: Blend all the ingredients. Pour the juice into a glass and garnish with the parsley leaf.

▸ Parsley, Spinach, Carrot, and Celery Juice:
Ingredients: 1 bunch of parsley, 1 bunch of spinach, 4 carrots, and 2 stalks of celery.
Preparation: Chop the parsley and spinach leaves and blend them along with the carrots and celery.

▸ Orange and Eggplant Juice:
Ingredients: 1 orange and half an eggplant.
Preparation: Add the peeled orange and half an eggplant with its peel, then blend, strain, and drink on an empty stomach.

▸ Pineapple, Celery, and Lemon Juice:
Ingredients: 1/4 tropical pineapple, 1/2 lemon, and 3 celery stalks.
Preparation: Peel and chop the pineapple, cut the lemon into quarters, and chop the celery into small strips. Blend all the ingredients.

MEDICINAL PLANTS

"The doctor of the future will be oneself" (Albert Schweitzer)

Since time immemorial, humanity has turned to the natural world for answers to its needs. Medicinal herbs, faithful companions on this journey, have generously shared their wisdom to ease ailments and enhance well-being. This ancient knowledge, carefully preserved through the ages, has found a renewed place in the modern world, offering a healthy and sustainable option to address today's challenges.

In a society increasingly conscious of the adverse effects of certain pharmaceutical treatments and the environmental toll of unsustainable practices, botanical remedies are experiencing a resurgence with renewed prominence. For those seeking a balanced, respectful lifestyle in harmony with the environment, these green treasures provide invaluable solutions. This revival not only reflects a growing interest in ecological approaches but also an evolution toward holistic care for both the body and the planet.

What makes these natural wonders truly extraordinary is the complexity of their compounds, capable of delivering antioxidant, anti-inflammatory, antibacterial, and antiviral properties, among others. Their potential ranges from alleviating everyday issues like sleeplessness or sluggish digestion to addressing conditions such as chronic stress or age-related ailments.

Beyond the ability to target specific concerns, these species serve as vital sources of micronutrients–vitamins, minerals, fiber, and antioxidants–that fortify the immune system and support long-term health. Incorporating them into dietary or self-care routines offers a simple, sustainable, and effective path toward illness prevention and enhanced overall wellness.

The botanical kingdom boasts remarkable diversity, featuring countless species uniquely suited to meet specific needs. Whether prepared as herbal teas, applied as balms or tinctures, or utilized in the form of essential oils, their applications are as versatile as they are effective, seamlessly fitting into various lifestyles.

More than mere remedies, these natural allies inspire us to reconnect with the world around us. Harnessing their benefits requires respect for environmental rhythms and a deeper appreciation for our planet's ecosystems. Each herb or extract serves as a tangible reminder of our connection to the living world, fostering a sense of harmony that transcends the physical and nurtures the spiritual.

In addition to their myriad health benefits, plant-based solutions stand out for their accessibility and practical versatility. Many species grow abundantly in wild habitats or can be easily cultivated in home gardens, offering an affordable, sustainable alternative. In a global context marked by economic inequalities, these wellness allies provide inclusive options to complement—or even replace—costly interventions.

Over the centuries, knowledge of these natural solutions has been carefully preserved through oral traditions and written records. This heritage, rooted in deep respect for biodiversity, has been bolstered by modern science, validating the effects of their active compounds and shedding light on their mechanisms of action. It represents a powerful synergy between tradition and innovation, broadening the therapeutic applications of these botanical marvels.

However, unlocking their full potential requires responsible use. Every human body is unique, and while these species possess well-documented therapeutic properties, they are not without risks. Misuse or interactions with conventional medications can lead to adverse effects. Therefore, obtaining accurate and reliable information is essential to ensure safe and effective usage.

One particularly fascinating aspect is how the components within a plant work in unison. Whole extracts, resulting from this intricate interaction, often produce more balanced and holistic effects compared to isolated compounds. Molecules interact in complementary ways, maximizing benefits while reducing potential side effects. Conversely, isolated active principles can provide concentrated solutions but may carry an increased risk of adverse effects on the body.

The innate harmony of these botanical wonders highlights one of biodiversity's greatest gifts—balance. Whole extracts are celebrated for their gentleness and ability to integrate seamlessly with the body's natural processes. On the other hand, synthesized compounds strive for potency, often at the expense of stability. The synergistic interaction between molecular components amplifies therapeutic benefits while limiting potential downsides, making them a choice deeply aligned with human needs.

Ultimately, medicinal plants transcend their role as therapeutic tools–they bridge ancestral wisdom and scientific innovation. They remind us that the health of our bodies and the well-being of our planet are profoundly interconnected. By safeguarding this invaluable legacy, we nurture not only our own health but also that of future generations, renewing the delicate balance between humanity and nature.

Essential Information

Although plants are natural in origin, they should not be considered entirely harmless. Their active compounds may cause adverse effects or trigger allergies in certain individuals.

Occasional consumption of an infusion is unlikely to cause harm. However, excessive, prolonged, or frequent use may result in discomfort, allergic reactions, or even toxicity.

Tolerance to natural remedies varies greatly among people. If you are pregnant, breastfeeding, or managing conditions such as chronic illnesses, allergies, kidney or liver insufficiency, cancer, or undergoing medical treatment, it is crucial to refer to the section titled "**Learn Everything You Need to Know About the Plants**" before using them. This section provides essential information on potential risks, contraindications, and interactions, enabling you to make informed and responsible decisions.

Guidelines for Care with Herbal Remedies

For best results, continue using the remedies until your symptoms have completely disappeared. The treatment duration will vary depending on factors like the severity of your condition, how it progresses, your personal commitment, and other important influences.

Keep in mind that some plants or herbal remedies are not suited for continuous or long-term use. In such cases, you will always find specific instructions that address this.

While following the guidelines for the remedies below, it is just as important to focus on the underlying causes of your symptoms. To better understand the root of your health concerns, I recommend referring to the first chapter of this book, specifically the section titled "Causes," where you'll discover essential insights into tackling the problem at its source.

Finally, remember that patience is vital. A condition that has lingered for months or years cannot be resolved in just a few days. Stay committed, persevere, and always prioritize your health and well-being.

Measurements

To achieve the best results when preparing infusions, decoctions, or other plant-based recipes, it is essential to follow these dosage guidelines:

- A tablespoon refers to a level tablespoon.
- A teaspoon refers to a level teaspoon.

Medicinal Plants for Hypertension

Medicinal plants offer an excellent way to naturally complement the management of hypertension. While all the options listed can help lower blood pressure, it is recommended to adopt a rotational approach: choose one or two plants to consume for three weeks, then switch to another two for the next three weeks. This method may help maximize benefits and prevent the body from developing tolerance.

For the best results, medicinal plants should be consumed in their natural form as infusions or decoctions, without adding sweeteners. However, if you prefer to sweeten your drink, it's advisable to use only 100% natural stevia as a healthy alternative.

Below, you will find a list of the most effective plants to help reduce blood pressure, along with preparation methods and recommended doses. Scientific names are included in parentheses, as these plants may be known by different names depending on the region or country.

Achicoria (Cichorium intybus)

Ingredients: 50 grams of dried chicory root and 1 liter of water.
Preparation: Boil the chicory root in a liter of water for 12 minutes. Remove from heat.
Dosage: Drink half a glass several times a day.

Cinnamon (Cinnamomum verum)

Ingredients: 1 or 2 tablespoons of cinnamon powder and 1 tablespoon of honey.
Preparation: Boil the cinnamon in water for 2 minutes and let it cool.
Dosage: Take it 3 or 4 times daily with a teaspoon of honey.

Hawthorn (Crataegus oxyacantha)

Ingredients: 2 teaspoons of hawthorn flowers. Water.
Preparation: Boil the equivalent of one cup of water. Add the flowers, cover, and let stand for 15 minutes; strain and drink.
Dosage: Drink 3 cups a day.

Horsetail (Equisetum arvense)

In decoction:
Ingredients: 4 tablespoons of dried plant in a liter and a half of water.
Preparation: Boil over low heat for 30 minutes. Let cool, filter, and drink.
Dosage: A cup in the morning and another at noon.
Observations: Avoid taking it after 6 pm due to its diuretic effect.

Infusion:
Ingredients: 2 to 4 tablespoons of horsetail per cup.
Preparation: Boil the water and let it steep for 5 minutes.
Dosage: Drink 3 cups a day.

Note: Horsetail should not be taken for more than 6 weeks at a time. Wait 2 months before using it again. If you take it for a prolonged period, supplement the treatment with potassium tablets.

Lavender (Lavandula angustifolia)

In decoction:
Ingredients: 1 to 2 teaspoons of dried lavender herb per cup of water.
Preparation: Boil the water, add the lavender, and leave it on the fire for 5 minutes. Turn off and let stand for another 3 minutes. Strain.
Dosage: Drink 2 or 3 cups a day. Taking it at night will also help you sleep.

Mistletoe (Viscum album)

Infusion:
Ingredients: 2 teaspoons of dried mistletoe leaves, 2 teaspoons of lemon balm leaves, and water.
Preparation: Put the mistletoe and lemon balm in a cup of boiling water and let it stand for 15 minutes.
Dosage: Drink the infusion in the morning and night for 15 days.

Decoction (with leaves):
Ingredients: 15 mistletoe leaves and water.
Preparation: Combine the mistletoe leaves and half a liter of water in a saucepan. Boil for 15 minutes, then turn off the heat, strain the mixture, and let it stand for 5 minutes.
Dosage: Consume the mixture in the morning and at night for 7 days.

Note: Do not take mistletoe for more than two months in a row. Take one month off for every two months of intake.

Olive Tree (Olea europaea)

Infusion:
Ingredients: 1 tablespoon of dried leaves and 250 ml of water.
Preparation: Boil the water, remove it from the heat, and add the tablespoon of olive leaves. Cover and let it stand for 10 minutes.
Dosage: Strain and drink two or three times a day.

Decoction:
Ingredients: 1 tablespoon of dried olive leaves or 20 grams of fresh leaves and 250 ml of water.
Preparation: Heat the water over the fire. When it starts to boil, add the olive leaves and let them cook for 5 minutes. Please turn off the heat and let them stand for 30 minutes.

Dosage: Strain and drink 2 or 3 times a day.

Note: Olive enhances vasodilator action, which is helpful, especially if you have minimal high blood pressure or find it difficult to reduce it. It is also beneficial in cases of stubborn hypertension.

Phytotherapy Recipes

While the plants mentioned above are effective when used individually, their benefits can be significantly enhanced when combined properly. Here are some especially effective combinations:

▸ **Phytotherapy Recipe No. 1**
Ingredients: 30 grams of olive leaves, 30 grams of hawthorn, 30 grams of sundew, 20 grams of mistletoe, and 20 grams of horsetail.
Preparation: Mix all the ingredients in a bowl. Add one teaspoon of the mixture to a cup of boiling water. Let it steep for 5 to 8 minutes. Strain and drink three times a day.

▸ **Phytotherapy Recipe No. 2**
Ingredients: 30 grams of olive leaves, 30 grams of hawthorn buckthorn, and 20 grams of lemon balm.
Preparation: Mix the ingredients in a bowl. Add one teaspoon of the mixture to a cup of boiling water. Let it steep for 5 to 8 minutes. Strain and drink three times a day.

▸ **Phytotherapy Recipe No. 3**
Ingredients: 5 grams of mistletoe, 10 grams of shepherd's purse, 20 grams of dandelion, 15 grams of horsetail, 10 grams of bloodroot, and 10 grams of yarrow.
Preparation: Mix all the ingredients in a bowl. Add one teaspoon of the mixture to a cup of boiling water. Let it steep for 5 to 8 minutes. Strain and drink three times a day.

Note: If your hypertension is emotionally driven, such as in cases of nervous or psychic hypertension, a soothing herbal infusion may provide significant relief. A blend of valerian, passionflower, hawthorn, and lavender, mixed in equal parts, has proven to be particularly effective.

For best results, I suggest consuming this infusion twice a day: once in the morning to promote a calm start to the day and again at night to encourage relaxation and restful sleep. This natural remedy can help address both the physical and emotional components of your hypertension.

Simple Steps to Make a Tincture for Hypertension

Tinctures, also known as concentrated botanical extracts, are an effective and potent way to harness the therapeutic benefits of medicinal plants. Through a careful extraction process, essential compounds, such as phytochemicals and active principles, are obtained, providing valuable healing properties.

These liquid solutions have been used for centuries in traditional medicine due to their proven efficacy and exceptional versatility. In recent years, they have regained their relevance thanks to the growing interest in natural remedies and herbal practices.

The method for preparing these extracts can vary, but it generally involves immersing plant parts—such as roots, leaves, flowers, or bark—in a solvent like alcohol, glycerin, or water. During the steeping process, the plant's active elements are extracted into the liquid, creating a medicinal concentrate that retains its essential properties.

One of the main advantages of these preparations is their practicality. They can be administered orally by adding a few drops to water or juice, allowing for rapid absorption. Additionally, their high concentration enables precise dosage adjustments based on individual needs.

▸ **Making an Olive Leaves Tincture:**

Ingredients: 50 dried olive leaves or 150 fresh leaves per liter of water.

Preparation: For fresh leaves, carefully clean them in water with baking soda for a few minutes. Wash and rinse well. Put the leaves in a pot with water and bring to a boil. Once it boils, lower the heat and simmer for 15 minutes. Remove the leaves, let them cool, strain, and pour the mixture into a glass bottle. Store this extract in the refrigerator.

Dosage: Take one teaspoon three times a day with meals. If the taste is too strong, dilute it with water.

Storage: Keep the tincture in a cool, dark place, and make sure to check the expiration date (1 year).

Learn Everything You Need to Know About the Plants

In this section, we'll delve into the most recommended botanical species for treating the condition at hand. You'll find essential information about their possible adverse effects, contraindications, and interactions, as well as detailed insights into each plant. From their descriptions and habitats to their uses, chemical components, histories, and therapeutic properties, this chapter is designed to take you on a fascinating journey of discovery.

My goal is to provide you with a comprehensive under-standing of these plants, helping you grasp their context and fully appreciate their many benefits. We'll explore their historical origins and significance in traditional medicine, highlighting their invaluable role in natural care.

I want you to become an expert on these species, capable of making informed decisions in your pursuit of wellness. Get ready to expand your knowledge and uncover the extraordinary healing power of nature!

Chicory (Cichorium intybus)

Description:
Chicory, scientifically known as Cichorium intybus, is a perennial herbaceous plant belonging to the Asteraceae family. Its erect, branched stem can reach a height of up to one meter. Its leaves are arranged as a basal rosette, lanceolate, and have a pronounced central vein. Chicory flowers are light blue and grouped in inflorescences as heads.

Habitat and Cultivation:
Chicory is native to Europe but is now distributed in many parts of the world. It prefers to grow in nutrient-rich, well-drained soils and can adapt to different climatic conditions. It is commonly found in meadows, roadsides, and vacant lots.

Parts Used:
Chicory is mainly grown for its roots, which are used for

various purposes. The roots are harvested in autumn after the plant has grown. The leaves and flowers are also used, although to a lesser extent.

Components:
This plant contains various active compounds, including sesquiterpenes, sesquiterpene lactones, inulin, tannins, flavonoids, and phenolic acids. These substances confer medicinal properties and health benefits.

History and Tradition:
The use of chicory dates back to ancient times. In ancient Egypt, it was used as food and to treat digestive problems. In the Middle Ages, chicory was cultivated in monasteries and used as a medicinal plant. Additionally, during coffee shortages in Europe, chicory root became a coffee substitute, especially during the war.

Therapeutic Properties:
Chicory has been traditionally used as a digestive tonic and hepatoprotective agent. It is attributed to diuretic, cholagogue, and mild laxative properties. Additionally, it is used in cases of liver and gallbladder disorders, such as jaundice and dyspepsia. The inulin in the plant also gives it prebiotic properties, promoting the growth of beneficial bacteria in the intestine.

Curiosities:
It is worth mentioning that roasted and ground chicory roots have been used as a substitute for coffee in some regions. This drink tastes similar to coffee but milder and slightly bitter. Chicory is also an ingredient in some alcoholic beverages, such as Angostura bitters.

Another interesting fact about chicory is that its flowers open and close in response to sunlight. During the day, the flowers open to attract pollinators, while at night, they close to protect pollen and prevent water loss.

Adverse or Side Effects:
Chicory may cause allergic reactions in some people, especially those sensitive to plants in the Asteraceae family. These reactions may include skin rashes, itching, or difficulty breathing. Additionally, excessive consumption may have a more pronounced laxative effect, which could cause diarrhea.

Contraindications:
It is recommended to avoid the consumption of chicory in

pregnant or breastfeeding women, as there is not enough scientific evidence on its safety in these situations. Also, people suffering from bile duct obstruction or gallstones should avoid consuming chicory, as it may stimulate bile production and worsen symptoms.

Interactions:
It is important to note that chicory may interact with certain medications used to treat clotting disorders, such as anticoagulants. The plant contains substances that could increase the risk of bleeding when combined with these drugs.

Cinnamon (Cinnamomum verum)

Description:
Cinnamon is an aromatic and flavorful spice obtained from the inner bark of trees belonging to Cinnamomum. There are several species of cinnamon trees, but the most common are Cinnamomum verum and Cinnamomum cassia. Cinnamon has a distinctive sweet odor and a warm, slightly spicy flavor.

Habitat and Cultivation:
Cinnamon is native to Sri Lanka but is also cultivated in other tropical regions of Asia, such as Indonesia, India, and Vietnam. Cinnamon trees prefer warm, humid climates at low to medium altitudes. They thrive in well-drained, nutrient-rich soils.

Parts Used:
The inner bark of cinnamon is used. To obtain it, the bark is peeled from the young branches of the cinnamon tree. The bark is extracted in thin strips and then rolled to form cinnamon sticks. Cinnamon can also be found in powdered form, which is obtained by grinding dried cinnamon sticks.

Components:
Cinnamon contains various elements that give flavor, aroma, and therapeutic properties. Essential oils, such as cinnamaldehyde, are the most prominent compounds responsible for cinnamon's distinctive aroma. It also contains eugenol, linalool, and coumarin, among other compounds.

History and Tradition:
Cinnamon has been appreciated for centuries. In ancient times, it was used as a spice, perfume, and medicine. It was considered

a treasure used in religious rituals and embalming practices. During the Middle Ages, cinnamon was highly valued in Europe and was one of the drivers of exploration and trade in search of new routes to cinnamon-producing regions.

Therapeutic Properties:
Cinnamon is attributed to antioxidant, anti-inflammatory, and antimicrobial properties. It has also been studied for its possible effects on regulating blood sugar and improving insulin sensitivity, which could benefit people with type 2 diabetes. Additionally, cinnamon may help improve digestion and relieve stomach upset.

Curiosities:
Historically, cinnamon has been used as an aphrodisiac. It was believed that its aroma and flavor could awaken sexual desire. Additionally, cinnamon has been considered a valuable spice and used as a currency of exchange in some ancient cultures.

Another interesting fact is that cinnamon has traditionally been used as an insect repellent. Its robust and spicy aroma helps keep mosquitoes and other pesky insects away. It can even be used as an essential oil to repel insects naturally.

Adverse or Side Effects:
Excessive consumption of cinnamon can cause mouth and digestive tract irritation. This is due to its high concentration of irritating compounds, such as cinnamaldehyde. Additionally, some people may be allergic to cinnamon and experience allergic reactions, such as skin rashes or difficulty breathing.

A potentially dangerous side effect of cinnamon is its coumarin content. Coumarin is a compound that can be toxic to the liver in high doses. However, the amount of coumarin in cinnamon varies depending on the species and how it is processed. Ceylon cinnamon (Cinnamomum verum) has lower coumarin levels than cassia cinnamon, which is more commonly found in the market.

Contraindications:
It is recommended to avoid consuming large quantities of cinnamon during pregnancy, as it may stimulate the uterus and increase the risk of miscarriage. Additionally, people with liver disease or coagulation disorders should be cautious when consuming cinnamon, as it may affect liver function and increase the risk of bleeding.

Interactions:

It may interact with some medications used to treat diabetes. It can potentiate the effects of these medications and decrease blood sugar levels, which can lead to hypoglycemia. Therefore, it is essential to monitor blood sugar levels closely and adjust the dosage of drugs in consultation with a physician.

Dandelion (Taraxacum officinale)

Description:
Dandelion, whose scientific name is Taraxacum officinale, is a perennial herbaceous plant in the Asteraceae family. It is a medium-sized plant that can grow to a height of 30 to 40 centimeters. It has toothed leaves that form a basal rosette at the base of the plant. Its bright yellow flowers are grouped in characteristic heads resembling tiny suns. After flowering, the flowers give way to a fluffy white seed head known as a "parachute, " quickly dispersed by the wind.

Habitat and Cultivation:
Dandelion is native to Europe and Asia but is now found worldwide. It is a very adaptable plant that can grow in various habitats, including meadows, gardens, fields, and roadsides. It is considered an invasive plant in some places because it can spread rapidly and displace other species. Regarding cultivation, dandelion is a hardy plant that can grow in almost any type of soil as long as it is well-drained. It can also grow in both full sun and partial shade areas.

Parts Used:
Dandelion leaves and roots are used for medicinal purposes. The young and tender leaves can be used in salads or cooked as vegetables. The roots are dried to make infusions, extracts, and tinctures.

Components:
It contains a variety of components beneficial to health. The leaves contain vitamins A, C, and K, as well as iron, calcium, and potassium minerals. The roots contain inulin, a type of soluble fiber, and phenolic compounds, flavonoids, and triterpenoids. These compounds are responsible for many of the therapeutic properties of dandelion.

History and Tradition:
Dandelion has been used in traditional medicine for centuries.

Its use dates back to ancient Greece and Rome, where it was used to treat digestive and liver problems. It has also been used in traditional Chinese and Ayurvedic medicine. In addition to its medicinal properties, dandelion also has a place in cultural tradition. For example, in some European cultures, blowing dandelion seeds is believed to bring good luck or fulfill wishes.

Therapeutic Properties:
Dandelion has many therapeutic properties that make it valuable in natural medicine. It has been traditionally used to stimulate digestion, relieve bloating and constipation, and promote liver and gallbladder health. In addition, dandelion has diuretic properties, which means it can help encourage the elimination of fluids and toxins from the body. It has also been used to promote kidney health and improve kidney function. Additionally, dandelion has antioxidant and anti-inflammatory properties, making it helpful in treating inflammatory conditions such as arthritis. However, it is essential to note that dandelion can interact with certain medications and may cause allergic reactions in some people.

Curiosities:
Dandelion has some exciting curiosities. One of them is its name, which comes from the French "dent de lion", which means "lion's tooth" in English. This is due to the shape of its leaves, which resemble the teeth of a lion. Another curiosity is that all parts of the dandelion are edible and have health benefits. Every part of the plant can be used in cooking or natural medicine, from the flowers to the roots. Additionally, dandelion is one of the first plants to bloom in spring, and its bright yellow flowers are a sign that winter is over and the growing season is in full swing.

Adverse or Side Effects:
Although dandelion is generally safe for most people, it may cause some adverse effects in some instances. The most common side effects include stomach upset, diarrhea, and allergic reactions in sensitive individuals. In addition, dandelion may have a diuretic effect, which can increase urine production. This can benefit some people, but can also lead to dehydration if insufficient fluid is consumed. Furthermore, excessive consumption of dandelion can interfere with certain medications, such as diuretics, so it is essential to use caution when combining it with other treatments.

Contraindications:
Although dandelion is considered safe for most people, there

are some contraindications to be aware of. People with known allergies to plants in the Asteraceae family, such as ragweed, chrysanthemum, or daisy, should avoid consuming dandelion, as they may have allergic reactions. Additionally, individuals with bile duct obstruction or gallstones should avoid dandelion consumption, as it may increase bile production and exacerbate these issues. If you have any specific health conditions, it is advisable to consult a healthcare professional before using dandelion.

Interactions:
It may interact with certain medications, so it is essential to exercise caution when combining it with other treatments. For example, dandelion may increase the effects of diuretic medications, which can lead to increased fluid and electrolyte removal from the body. Additionally, dandelions may interact with drugs metabolized in the liver, such as blood thinners, diabetes medications, and cholesterol medications. This can affect the effectiveness and safety of these medications. If you are taking any medications, it is advisable to consult your doctor before using dandelion or supplements containing dandelion.

Hawthorn (Crataegus monogyna)

Description:
Hawthorn is a shrub or small tree belonging to the Rosaceae family, with the scientific name Crataegus monogyna. Native to Europe, it is also found in other parts of the world. The hawthorn features a short trunk and thorny branches with toothed, lance-shaped leaves. It produces small white flowers in spring with five petals and a delicate aroma. These flowers transform into small red or black berries in the fall.

Habitat and cultivation:
Hawthorn thrives in various habitats, including woodlands, scrub, hedgerows, and grasslands. It is a very hardy plant that can adapt to different types of soils, although it prefers well-drained, slightly acidic soils. It can grow in both full sun and partial shade. Due to its decorative flowers and showy berries, hawthorn is widely cultivated as an ornamental plant in gardens and parks.

Parts used:
The hawthorn's flowers, leaves, and berries are used for

medicinal purposes. The flowers are harvested in spring before they open fully, the leaves are collected in spring or summer, and the berries are harvested in autumn.

Components:
Hawthorn contains various health-promoting constituents. The flowers contain flavonoids, tannins, and essential oils. The leaves also contain flavonoids, organic acids, and vitamin C. The berries are rich in vitamin C and also contain flavonoids and antioxidants.

History and tradition:
Hawthorn has a long history of use in traditional European medicine. It has been used for centuries to treat heart and circulatory problems like heart failure and hypertension. Additionally, it has been used to relieve anxiety, improve sleep, and promote digestion. In some European cultures, it has also been considered a symbol of protection and good luck.

Therapeutic properties:
Hawthorn has therapeutic properties that make it valuable in natural medicine. It has been used to improve cardiovascular health and promote blood circulation, helping to strengthen the heart muscle, regulate heart rhythm, and lower blood pressure. It has also been used to relieve symptoms of heart failure, such as fatigue, shortness of breath, and swelling. Moreover, hawthorn has antioxidant and anti-inflammatory properties, which can help protect cells from oxidative damage and reduce inflammation. It has also been used to relieve anxiety, improve sleep quality, and promote healthy digestion.

Curiosities:
Hawthorn has some exciting aspects. One is its long history of use in traditional European medicine as a natural remedy for heart and circulatory problems. In addition, hawthorn is known for its delicate white flowers and red or black berries, which give it a striking and attractive appearance in gardens and parks. Another interesting fact is that in some European cultures, the hawthorn symbolizes protection and good luck, which are associated with strength and longevity.

Adverse or side effects:
Although hawthorn is generally safe for most people, it may cause some adverse effects in some instances. The most common side effects include stomach upset, nausea, diarrhea, and headaches. Additionally, on rare occasions, hawthorn may trigger an allergic reaction in sensitive individuals. Excessive

consumption of hawthorn has also been reported to cause a significant lowering of blood pressure, which can be dangerous for those with already low blood pressure. Therefore, it is essential to use it cautiously and consult a healthcare professional if adverse effects are experienced.

Contraindications:
Although hawthorn is generally safe, there are some contraindications to consider. People taking blood pressure medications, blood thinners, or heart medications should exercise caution when using hawthorn, as it may interact with these drugs and potentially alter their effects. Pregnant or nursing women should avoid using hawthorn due to the lack of evidence regarding its safety during these stages. If you have any specific health conditions or are taking any medications, it is advisable to consult a healthcare professional before using hawthorn.

Interactions:
It may interact with certain medications, so it is essential to use caution when combining it with other treatments. It may enhance the effects of blood pressure medications, such as beta-blockers and angiotensin-converting enzyme inhibitors, potentially causing excessive blood pressure lowering. It may also interact with blood-thinning medications, such as warfarin, increasing the risk of bleeding. Additionally, hawthorn may interfere with the absorption of certain medications, such as calcium channel blockers. Therefore, it is essential to inform your doctor if you are taking hawthorn or supplements containing hawthorn so they can evaluate possible interactions and adjust treatments accordingly.

Horsetail (Equisetum arvense)

Description:
Horsetail is a perennial plant belonging to the genus Equisetum. It is characterized by hollow, jointed stems that resemble horse tails. It has small leaves and cone-shaped spores at the top of the stems.

Habitat and Cultivation:
Horsetail is commonly found in wet and marshy areas worldwide. It grows in mineral-rich soils and can tolerate different light and water conditions. It can be grown in gardens

and is also found in the wild.

Parts Used:
The parts used of horsetail are the sterile stems that grow in spring before the appearance of spores. These stems are harvested and used fresh and dried to obtain their medicinal properties.

Components:
Horsetail contains several beneficial constituents, including silica, flavonoids, minerals (such as potassium and calcium), ascorbic acid (vitamin C), and alkaloids. Silica is a main component contributing to the plant's healing properties.

History and Tradition:
Horsetail (Equisetum arvense) has been used in traditional medicine for centuries due to its medicinal properties and health benefits. It is a perennial plant in various parts of the world, including Europe, Asia, and North America. Its name comes from its appearance, as its stems resemble horse tails.

This plant has been valued in the history and traditions of different cultures. In ancient Rome, for example, it was believed to have healing properties and was used to treat wounds and urinary problems. It was also used to treat various ailments in Traditional Chinese Medicine and Indian Ayurvedic medicine.

In addition to its medicinal uses, horsetail has also been used in agriculture and gardening due to its silica content, which strengthens plant tissues and promotes plant growth. It has also been used in cosmetic products and in the textile industry to enhance fabric fibers.

Therapeutic Properties:
Horsetail is known for its therapeutic properties and health benefits. Some of its most outstanding properties are:

Natural Diuretic: Horsetail has a mild diuretic effect, stimulating urine production and helping eliminate toxins and wastes from the body. This can be beneficial in treating fluid retention, reducing swelling, and promoting kidney health.

Strengthening Bone and Tissue: Horsetail contains silica, a mineral in high concentrations in this plant. Silica is essential for forming and strengthening connective tissues, such as bones, cartilage, and nails. It can also help promote healthy skin, hair, and teeth.

Anti-inflammatory Properties: Horsetail has anti-inflammatory properties, which can help reduce inflammation in the body. This can be beneficial in treating inflammatory conditions such as arthritis and inflammatory bowel disease.

Improving Urinary System Health: Horsetail has traditionally been used to treat urinary system conditions, such as urinary tract infections and kidney stones. Its diuretic effect can help cleanse and detoxify the kidneys, thus promoting kidney health and preventing stone formation.

Antioxidant Action: Horsetail contains antioxidants that help protect cells from damage caused by free radicals. Free radicals are unstable molecules that can damage DNA and contribute to aging and various diseases. The antioxidants in horsetail help neutralize these free radicals and protect the body against oxidative stress.

Horsetail can be consumed as an infusion, capsule, or liquid extract.

Curiosities:
Horsetail is a perennial herb that grows worldwide in wet, marshy areas. It receives its name because of its distinctive appearance, resembling a horsetail's bristles. In addition to its peculiar appearance, horsetail has several interesting curio-sities:

Living Fossils: Horsetails are considered living fossils, as they are plants that have existed on Earth for millions of years. The first horsetail species are said to have emerged more than 300 million years ago, during the Carboniferous period.

Silica Content: It is one of the few plants that contains high levels of silica, an essential mineral component for human health. This makes it a popular plant in traditional medicine for strengthening hair, nails, and bones.

Use in Gardening: Horsetail is appreciated in gardening besides its medicinal properties. Its hollow, jointed stems give it a unique structure, and it is often used as an ornamental plant in water gardens or to create natural borders in flower beds.

Adverse or Side Effects:
Despite its potential benefits, horsetail may have some adverse effects. Some of them are:

Thiaminase Toxicity: Horsetail contains an enzyme called

thiaminase, which can interfere with the absorption of vitamin B1 (thiamine). This can lead to thiamine deficiency in the body if consumed in large amounts or for prolonged periods.

Interference with Medications: Horsetail may interact with certain medications, such as diuretics or blood thinners. If you take any medication, consult a physician before using the plant to avoid negative interactions.

Allergic Reactions: Some people may be allergic to horsetail. This allergy may manifest as rashes, itching, swelling, or difficulty breathing. If you experience any allergic reaction, seek immediate medical attention.

Contraindications:
There are contraindications to be aware of when using horsetail:

Pregnancy and Lactation: The safety of horsetail during pregnancy and lactation has not been sufficiently investigated. As a precaution, it is recommended that pregnant or nursing women avoid use or consult a physician before use.

Kidney Problems: Due to its silica content and diuretic capacity, caution is advised in people with kidney problems, such as kidney stones or kidney failure, as horsetail may aggravate these conditions.

Interactions:
Horsetail may interact with certain medications and supplements, so it is essential to use caution when combining it with other treatments. Some known interactions include:

Diuretic Medications: Horsetail has natural diuretic properties to increase the diuretic effect of diuretic medications. This could lead to excessive fluid and mineral loss in the body.

Anticoagulants: It may have mild anticoagulant effects, which could increase the risk of bleeding when combined with anticoagulant medications such as warfarin. Medical supervision is recommended if both treatments are used.

Lavender (Lavandula angustifolia)

Description:
Lavender, also known as Lavandula, is a perennial plant of the Lamiaceae family characterized by its fragrant violet or lavender flowers. Originally native to the Mediterranean region, lavender is now cultivated worldwide for its aromatic and therapeutic properties. It is a medium-sized plant with narrow, lanceolate leaves and branched stems. The plant's most distinctive and widely used part is its flowers, which appear in long, slender spikes.

Habitat and cultivation:
Lavender thrives in sunny, dry areas and prefers well-drained soils, as it does not tolerate excess moisture. It is commonly grown in Mediterranean climates and has also adapted successfully to regions such as southern France, England, and the United States. Lavender is a hardy plant that adapts well to different climatic conditions. It is propagated by seed or cuttings and can be grown in gardens and pots.

Parts used:
The primary part is its flowers, which are harvested in full bloom and dried for later use. Although the leaves and stems can also be utilized, the flowers are the most valued due to their aroma and therapeutic properties. Lavender also produces essential oil extracted from the flowers by steam distillation.

Components:
Lavender contains various constituents that give it its aroma and therapeutic properties. Key elements include essential oils such as linalool and linalyl acetate, which are responsible for its characteristic fragrance. It also contains compounds like cineol, geraniol, and limonene. These components provide relaxing, anti-inflammatory, analgesic, and antiseptic properties.

History and tradition:
The name Lavender derives from the Latin "lavare", meaning "to wash". The Romans used lavender in their baths and as a perfume. During the Middle Ages, lavender was a natural remedy for various ailments and diseases. It was also used to scent clothes and repel insects. Today, lavender is widely used in the cosmetic industry, aromatherapy, and herbal medicine.

Therapeutic properties:

Lavender is known for its relaxing and calming effects. It is commonly used to relieve stress, anxiety, and insomnia. The scent of lavender has a sedative effect and can help induce sleep and improve the quality of rest. Additionally, lavender has anti-inflammatory and analgesic properties, making it helpful in relieving muscle and joint pain. Due to its antiseptic properties it has also been used to treat skin problems such as burns, wounds, and insect bites. Lavender essential oil is employed in massages, relaxing baths, inhalations, and cosmetic products and perfumes.

Curiosities:
It is one of the most widely used plants in aromatherapy due to its relaxing aroma. Its soft and floral fragrance is associated with calmness and relaxation, making it popular in bath and personal care products, as well as in air fresheners and scented candles.

Another interesting tidbit is that lavender has traditionally been used as an insect repellent. Its strong, distinctive scent helps keep mosquitoes and other pesky insects away. Additionally, lavender can be used to repel moths and protect clothing from damage caused by these insects.

Adverse or side effects:
Lavender is considered safe when used correctly. However, some people may be allergic and experience reactions such as skin rashes, swelling, or difficulty breathing. Therefore, it is essential to perform a patch test before using lavender-containing products on the skin.

In rare cases, topical lavender essential oil may cause skin irritation, mainly if used in high concentrations or undiluted. It is crucial to dilute the essential oil before application and avoid direct contact with the eyes and mucous membranes.

Contraindications:
It is recommended to avoid the use of lavender during pregnancy, as it may stimulate the uterus and increase the risk of miscarriage. Additionally, caution should be exercised by individuals sensitive to the components of lavender, as they may experience allergic reactions.

Interactions:
It is important to note that lavender essential oil may interact with certain sedative or central nervous system depressant drugs, such as barbiturates and tranquilizers. Lavender may potentiate the sedative effects of these drugs, potentially causing excessive drowsiness or difficulty concentrating.

Lemon Balm (Melissa officinalis)

Description:
Lemon balm, scientifically known as Melissa officinalis, is a perennial herbaceous plant from the Lamiaceae family. It is characterized by its oval, toothed, light green leaves with a delightful citrus aroma. The plant reaches a height of approximately 60-90 cm and produces small white or yellow flowers in clusters.

Habitat and cultivation:
Lemon balm is native to the Mediterranean region but is now cultivated in various parts of the world due to its medicinal properties and use in the cosmetic and culinary industries. It prefers rich, well-drained soils and adapts to different climates, from warm to cold. It is relatively easy to grow and can be found in gardens and commercial cultivation.

Parts used:
The primary parts used are the leaves and flowers. The leaves are harvested and dried for later use, but they can also be used fresh in infusions, salads, and culinary dishes. The flowers of lemon balm have a milder aroma and are used to a lesser extent, but they can also be collected and dried together with the leaves.

Components:
Among the main components are essential oils such as citronellal, citral, and geraniol, which give it its characteristic citrus aroma. It also contains phenolic acids, flavonoids, and tannins, which provide antioxidant and anti-inflammatory properties.

History and tradition:
The name "Melissa" is said to come from ancient Greek and means "bee", as bees are attracted to its sweet fragrance. In ancient Greece, physicians and philosophers such as Hippocrates and Dioscorides recommended lemon balm to treat various ailments, including digestive disorders, insomnia, and anxiety. Additionally, lemon balm was used as a sacred plant in religious rituals and was believed to have properties to attract love and happiness.

Therapeutic properties:
Lemon balm has been shown to have calming and relaxing effects. It is commonly used to relieve stress, anxiety, and

insomnia. It also has digestive properties and treats problems such as upset stomach, intestinal spasms, and indigestion. Moreover, it has been employed to relieve cold symptoms such as nasal congestion and fever. Due to its antiviral and soothing properties, topical use of lemon balm may also be beneficial in treating skin conditions such as cold sores and insect bites.

Curiosities:
There are several interesting aspects to note. For example, it is believed that the name "Melissa" comes from ancient Greek and means "bee. " Bees are attracted to lemon balm's sweet fragrance and often visit its flowers. This makes lemon balm a highly prized plant in gardens, as it brings beauty and attracts these essential pollinators.

Another curiosity is that lemon balm has historically been used as a medicinal plant and culinary ingredient. In ancient Greece, it was used to treat various disorders and ailments. Additionally, its fresh or dried leaves have been used in cooking as a condiment, adding a citrusy and refreshing flavor to sweet and savory dishes and hot and cold drinks.

Adverse or side effects:
Lemon balm is generally considered a safe plant when used correctly. However, some people may be allergic to it and experience reactions such as skin rashes, itching, or swelling. Therefore, performing a sensitivity test before using lemon balm products is essential.

In rare cases, excessive consumption of lemon balm may cause side effects such as headache, dizziness, nausea, or stomach irritation. Moreover, high doses of lemon balm can have a sedative effect, so it is recommended to avoid excessive consumption or combining it with sedative drugs.

Contraindications:
It should not be used during pregnancy and lactation, as insufficient scientific evidence guarantees its safety in these stages. Additionally, caution should be exercised in people with hypothyroidism, as it may interfere with thyroid function.

Caution is also advised for people about to undergo surgery, as lemon balm may have sedative effects and interact with anesthetic drugs. It is recommended that they discontinue using lemon balm at least two weeks before any surgical procedure.

Interactions:

Lemon balm has been observed to enhance the sedative effects of drugs that act on the central nervous system, such as tranquilizers, antidepressants, or hypnotics. Therefore, it is essential to be cautious when combining lemon balm with these drugs, as it may increase drowsiness or cause a lack of concentration.

Additionally, it may interact with anticoagulant drugs, such as warfarin, and increase the risk of bleeding. Therefore, you should consult a doctor before using lemon balm products if taking any anticoagulant medication.

Mistletoe (Viscum album)

Description:
Mistletoe is a perennial, hemiparasitic plant belonging to the Santalaceae family. There are different species of mistletoe, but the best-known is the European mistletoe or Viscum album. It has woody, flexible stems that form a rounded structure. The leaves are small and yellowish-green. The small, white, or pale yellow flowers are grouped in clusters. Mistletoe produces white, sticky berries that are toxic to humans but serve as an essential food source for birds.

Habitat and cultivation:
Mistletoe is found worldwide but is most common in temperate northern hemisphere regions, such as Europe and North America. It grows mainly on deciduous trees like oaks, apples, willows, and pines. Mistletoe is a hemiparasitic plant that obtains part of its nutrients from its host. Although it can grow wild, it is also cultivated commercially for use in herbal medicine and traditional festivals.

Parts used:
Mistletoe's leaves and stems are used for medicinal purposes. They are harvested mainly in winter when the plant is resting. The berries are also used in specific preparations, but are toxic and should be handled cautiously.

Components:
Mistletoe contains a variety of chemical compounds that give it its therapeutic properties. The most critical components include lectins, polyphenols, flavonoids, triterpenoids and lignans. These compounds have antioxidant, anti-inflammatory, and anti-tumor

properties, among other beneficial health effects.

History and tradition:
Mistletoe has a long history and tradition associated with its use in medicine and festivities. In ancient Greece and Rome, it was considered a sacred plant and was believed to have healing and protective properties. The Celtic Druids also used mistletoe in their religious rituals and considered it a magical plant with healing and protective powers against evil spirits. Today, mistletoe has become a symbol of good luck and love in many cultures, especially during the Christmas season, when it is hung on the doorsteps of homes and used for kissing underneath.

Therapeutic properties:
Mistletoe has been used in traditional herbal medicine to treat various health conditions. It has been used as a remedy for high blood pressure, cardiovascular disease, nervous system disorders, immunomodulation, and cancer. Compounds in mistletoe have anti-tumor properties and may help inhibit the growth and spread of cancer cells. However, it is essential to note that a healthcare professional should supervise the use of mistletoe, as it can have side effects and contraindications, especially at high doses. Additionally, mistletoe can interact with certain medications, such as anticoagulants, so caution is advised when combining it with other treatments.

Curiosities:
Mistletoe's history and use have some interesting curiosities associated with it. One of the most well-known is its association with Christmas. In many European and North American cultures, hanging a sprig of mistletoe on the door or ceiling during Christmas symbolizes good luck and love.

Adverse effects:
Although it has been used in herbal medicine for centuries, it may have adverse side effects in some individuals. Consuming mistletoe in large quantities or without proper medical supervision may cause nausea, vomiting, diarrhea, and stomach upset. Additionally, mistletoe berries are toxic and can cause more severe symptoms, such as difficulty breathing, irregular heartbeat, and seizures. Therefore, it is essential to exercise caution and avoid consuming mistletoe berries.

Contraindications:
Mistletoe is sometimes contraindicated, and it is essential to be aware of this before using it for medicinal purposes. Pregnant or lactating women should avoid consuming mistletoe, as it may

affect hormonal dynamics and potentially adversely affect pregnancy and lactation. Additionally, mistletoe may interact with certain medications, such as anticoagulants, so individuals taking such medications should avoid it or use it only under the supervision of a healthcare professional.

Interactions:
It may interact with certain medications, potentially altering their effectiveness or increasing the risk of adverse effects. For example, mistletoe may increase the risk of bleeding in individuals taking anticoagulants or antiplatelet drugs, such as warfarin or aspirin. It has also been observed that mistletoe may interact with medications used to treat diabetes, lowering blood sugar levels. Therefore, informing your doctor if you are using mistletoe as part of your treatment is essential, and evaluating any possible interactions is necessary.

Olive Tree (Olea europaea)

Description:
Olive leaves are the foliage of the olive tree, scientifically known as Olea europaea. These leaves are elongated and lanceolate in shape, silvery-green on top and lighter on the underside. They have a smooth texture and are arranged opposite each other on the stem. Olive leaves are known for their characteristic aroma and for containing several com-pounds beneficial to health.

Habitat and cultivation:
The olive tree is native to the Mediterranean region but is now cultivated in various parts of the world. It requires a warm, sunny climate to grow properly. Olive trees are mainly found in Mediterranean areas, such as Spain, Italy, Greece, and southern France. Olive cultivation is an essential agricultural activity in these regions, as olives are used for olive oil production and consumption.

Parts used:
The leaves are mainly used for medicinal purposes. They are generally harvested during the olive harvest season, as they have a higher content of beneficial compounds. The leaves are dried to make infusions or extracts, which are then consumed as natural supplements.

Components:

Olive leaves contain various beneficial compounds, the most important of which is oleuropein. This polyphenol has antioxidant, anti-inflammatory, and antimicrobial properties. Additionally, olive leaves contain flavonoids, triterpenes, and phenolic acids, which contribute to their therapeutic properties.

History and tradition:
The olive tree has been cultivated and used since ancient times. Olive oil and olives have been part of the Mediterranean diet and are considered sources of health and longevity. Olive leaves have also been used in traditional medicine for centuries, especially in the folk medicine of Mediterranean countries such as Spain and Italy. In ancient Greece, olive leaves were considered symbols of peace and victory and were given as prizes to winning athletes in the Olympic Games.

Therapeutic properties:
Olive leaves have been used in traditional herbal medicine for their therapeutic properties. Compounds present in olive leaves have been shown to have antioxidant, anti-inflammatory, hypotensive, and antimicrobial effects. They have been used as natural supplements to support cardiovascular health, reduce blood pressure, enhance the immune system, and fight free radicals. Olive leaves have also been studied for their potential anti-cancer and anti-diabetic effects.

Curiosities:
Olive leaves have some interesting curiosities associated with their history and use. One curiosity is that the olive tree is considered one of the oldest trees cultivated by humans, with evidence of its cultivation dating back over 6,000 years. Additionally, the olive tree symbolizes resilience and longevity, as it can survive in adverse conditions and live for centuries. It is also interesting to note that olive oil, obtained from the olives of the olive tree, is known as "liquid gold" due to its nutritional value and health benefits.

Adverse or side effects:
Although olive leaves are generally considered safe for consumption, some may experience adverse side effects. Excessive consumption may cause stomach upset, diarrhea, or nausea. Additionally, some people may be allergic to olive tree pollen, which can cause symptoms such as sneezing, itchy eyes, and nasal congestion. If adverse effects are experienced, it is essential to use caution and discontinue the use of olive leaves.

Contraindications:

Although olive leaves are considered safe for most people, there are some essential contraindications to be aware of. Pregnant or nursing women should avoid consuming olive leaves, as not enough studies have been conducted on their safety in these groups. Additionally, people taking medications for high blood pressure should use caution when consuming olive leaves, as they may interact with these medications and potentially cause excessive blood pressure lowering.

Interactions:
Olive leaves may interact with certain medications, potentially affecting their effectiveness or causing adverse effects. For example, olive leaves may increase the impact of anticoagulant drugs, such as warfarin, raising the risk of bleeding. Additionally, olive leaves may interact with antihypertensive medications, potentially causing excessive blood pressure lowering. It has also been observed that olive leaves may interact with diabetes medications, as they may lower blood sugar levels. Therefore, informing your doctor if you are using olive leaves as part of your treatment is essential, as well as evaluating any possible interactions.

Passionflower (Passiflora incarnata)

Description:
Passionflower, whose scientific name is Passiflora incarnata, is a perennial climbing plant belonging to the Passifloraceae family. It is characterized by its beautiful, exotic flowers and edible fruits. Passionflower flowers are large, peculiarly shaped, and showy, with white or pink petals and a crown of colorful filaments in the center. The leaves are green and divided into several lobes. The plant can reach a height of up to 5 meters and spread along supporting structures, such as walls or fences.

Habitat and cultivation:
Passionflower is native to South and Central America but is now found in various tropical and subtropical regions worldwide. It grows wild in forests, riverbanks, and disturbed areas. As for cultivation, passionflower can be grown in warm, humid climates, preferably in well-drained, fertile soils. It can also be grown in pots indoors, provided it is given sufficient light and humidity.

Parts used:

The leaves and flowers are mainly used. The leaves are collected and dried for later use as tea, liquid extract, or capsules. The flowers can also be dried and used in herbal preparations. In some cases, passionflower fruits are also used for culinary purposes, as they are edible and have a sweet and juicy flavor.

Components:
The main components are alkaloids, such as harmine and harmaline, which have sedative and anxiolytic properties. The plant also contains flavonoids, such as quercetin and kaempferol, which have antioxidant and anti-inflammatory properties.

History and tradition:
Passionflower has a long history of use in traditional medicine. Native Americans reportedly used it to treat various disorders, such as insomnia, anxiety, and upset stomachs. In addition, in some cultures, passionflower is used as a sacred plant in rituals and ceremonies.

Therapeutic properties:
It has been shown to have sedative and anxiolytic effects, making it a natural choice for relieving stress, anxiety, and sleep disorders. It has also been used to alleviate menopausal symptoms, such as hot flashes and irritability. In addition, passionflower has antispasmodic properties, making it helpful in relieving menstrual cramps and stomach pains. Some studies also suggest that passionflower may have neuroprotective properties and help improve memory and concentration.

Curiosities:
There are several interesting aspects to highlight. For example, the plant's name, passionflower, comes from the Latin "passio" (passion) and "flora" (flower), referring to its exuberant and showy flowering. Passionflower flowers are considered a masterpiece of nature, with a complex structure and unique beauty that has captured the attention of botanists and plant lovers for centuries.

Another curiosity is that the passionflower is Paraguay's national flower, known as "mburucuyá". In addition, in some Latin American countries, it is used to make refreshing drinks and traditional desserts, such as "maracuya" in Brazil.

Adverse or side effects:
It is generally considered a safe plant when used correctly. However, in rare cases, some people may experience mild side

effects such as drowsiness, dizziness, or stomach upset. These side effects are usually temporary and disappear once the plant is discontinued.

Additionally, it has been observed that high doses of passionflower may have a more potent sedative effect, so it is recommended to avoid excessive consumption or combining it with sedative drugs, as it may increase the sedative effects and cause excessive drowsiness.

Contraindications:
It is recommended to avoid the use of passionflower during pregnancy and lactation, as there is not enough scientific evidence to guarantee its safety during these stages. Additionally, caution should be exercised in individuals with liver or kidney disease, as some studies suggest that passionflower may affect these organ functions.

Caution is also advised for individuals who are about to undergo surgery, as passionflower may have sedative effects and could interact with anesthetic medications. It is recommended that passionflower be discontinued at least two weeks before any surgical procedure.

Interactions:
It has been observed that passionflower can enhance the sedative effects of drugs that act on the central nervous system, such as tranquilizers, antidepressants, or hypnotics. Therefore, it is essential to be cautious when combining passionflower with these drugs, as it may increase drowsiness or impair concentration.

Additionally, it may interact with blood-thinning medications, such as warfarin, and increase the risk of bleeding. Therefore, you should consult a physician before using passionflower products if you take any anticoagulant medication.

Valerian (Valeriana officinalis)

Description:
Valerian, whose scientific name is Valeriana officinalis, is a perennial herbaceous plant in the Valerianaceae family. It is characterized by its erect stems, compound leaves, and small white or pink flowers grouped in inflorescences. The leaves are

opposite and feathery, while the flowers are small and fragrant. The plant can reach a height of up to 1 meter and has a characteristic, somewhat unpleasant odor that intensifies when dried.

Habitat and cultivation:

Valerian is native to Europe and Asia but is now found in various regions worldwide. It grows wild in wet meadows, forests, and riverbanks. Cultivation can be grown in temperate and cool climates, preferably in well-drained, nutrient-rich soils. It is propagated by seed or root division and requires care and patience, as it can take several years to reach total growth and develop its medicinal properties.

Parts used:

Valerian roots are primarily used, along with the aerial parts of the plant, such as leaves and stems, to a lesser extent. The roots are harvested and dried for later use in herbal preparations. Valerian roots are thick and fibrous and have a strong, characteristic aroma. The aerial parts can also be used fresh or dried, but generally contain a lower concentration of the active compounds.

Components:

Among the main components are valerenoids, volatile compounds with sedative and anxiolytic effects. It also contains essential oils, such as valerianic acid and borneol, which contribute to its characteristic aroma and have relaxing and calming properties.

History and tradition:

Valerian has a long history of use in traditional medicine. For example, the ancient Greeks and Romans used it to treat sleep disorders, anxiety, and digestive problems. Traditional Chinese medicine has been used for centuries to treat insomnia, agitation, and headaches.

Over the years, Valerian has been the subject of numerous legends and superstitions. It was said to have magical properties and was used to ward off evil spirits and protect against witchcraft. Planting Valerian near a house was even believed to attract love and happiness.

Therapeutic properties:

Valerian has been shown to have sedative, calming, and relaxing effects. It is used primarily as a sleep aid and improves sleep quality, especially in mild to moderate insomnia. It has also been used to relieve anxiety, stress, and depression symptoms. Additionally, it can help relieve headaches, muscle spasms, and digestive problems such as indigestion and colic.

Curiosities:
There are some exciting aspects worth noting. For example, the name "valerian" comes from the Latin "valere", which means "to be healthy" or "to have strength". This is because the plant has been used for centuries for its medicinal properties to promote relaxation and well-being.

Another curiosity is that valerian has been used as a natural insect repellent since ancient times. Its strong and characteristic aroma was believed to keep mosquitoes and other undesirable insects away, so valerian branches were placed on windows and doors to protect against bites.

In addition, valerian is a very attractive plant for cats. Some felines are susceptible to its scent and may be very interested in the roots or aerial parts of the plant. Cats have been observed to rub themselves against valerian, bite it, or play with it, which gives them great excitement and joy. For this reason, valerian is also known as "catnip".

Adverse effects:
Valerian is generally considered safe when used correctly. However, some people may experience mild side effects, such as drowsiness, dizziness, headache, or upset stomach. These side effects are usually temporary and disappear once the plant is discontinued.

Rare allergic reactions to valerian have been reported. These reactions may manifest as skin rashes, itching, or difficulty breathing. If these symptoms occur, discontinue valerian use and seek medical attention immediately.

Contraindications:
Valerian should not be used during pregnancy and lactation, as insufficient scientific evidence guarantees its safety during these stages. Additionally, caution should be exercised in people with liver or kidney disease, as some studies suggest that Valerian may affect these organ functions.

It is also recommended to avoid excessive valerian consumption, as it may cause excessive drowsiness and difficulty concentrating. Caution should be exercised when driving or operating machinery after taking valerian, as it may affect one's reaction ability.

Interactions:
It has been observed that valerian can enhance the sedative effects of drugs that act on the central nervous system, such as tranquilizers, antidepressants, or hypnotics. Therefore, it is essential to be cautious when combining valerian with these drugs, as it may increase drowsiness or impair concentration.

Additionally, it may interact with metabolized medications in the liver, such as blood thinners, anticonvulsants, or cancer drugs. It may affect how the body processes these drugs, potentially altering their effectiveness or increasing side effects.

FINAL NOTE

Thank you very much for choosing this book to accompany you on your path to complete health. If you find the information, advice, or remedies I share here useful, would you do me a favor? Taking a moment to leave your review or rating (several stars would be greatly appreciated) is an incredible way to help me continue creating valuable content while also guiding others who, like you, are seeking to improve their health and well-being. Thank you so much for being part of this wellness community!

With gratitude,

                              Isabel

Important Note on Printing and Shipping:
All of my paperback books are printed and distributed exclusively by Amazon and its affiliated printing facilities. If you encounter any issues with print quality or delivery, please contact Amazon Customer Service directly for assistance.

As the author, I have no control over these processes, so I kindly request that your reviews focus solely on the content, remedies, or information within this work. Some readers leave negative ratings due to shipping or binding issues, unaware that these matters are, unfortunately, entirely beyond my control and ability to resolve. Thank you from the bottom of my heart for your understanding!

AUTHOR'S BOOKS

- **ACID REFLUX**. Foods, Supplements & Medicinal Plants
- **ALLERGIES**. Foods, Supplements & Herbs
- **ANXIETY**. Foods, Supplements & Herbs
- **ARTHRITIS**. Foods, Supplements & Medicinal Plants
- **CHOLESTEROL**. Foods, Supplements & Medicinal Plants
- **DIABETES**. Foods, Supplements & Herbs
- **CONSTIPATION**. Foods, Supplements & Herbs
- **FIBROMYALGIA**. Foods, Supplements & Medicinal Plants
- **GASTRITIS**. Foods, Supplements & Herbs
- **HEMORRHOIDS**. Foods, Supplements & Herbs
- **HYPERTENSION**. Foods, Supplements & Medicinal Plants
- **INSOMNIA**. Foods, Supplements & Herbs
- **MENOPAUSE**. Foods, Supplements & Medicinal Plants
- **OSTEOARTHRITIS**. Foods, Supplements & Herbs
- **SIBO**. Foods, Supplements & Medicinal Plants
- **VARICOSE VEINS**. Foods, Supplements & Herbs

Roots that Inspire: From Obstacles to New Horizons

Born in 1971 in Gáldar, Gran Canaria, Isabel grew up in an environment steeped in tradition and ancestral wisdom. Surrounded by the knowledge of her homeland, she learned from an early age to appreciate the healing power of medicinal plants, home remedies, and the importance of nutrition as foundations for nurturing both body and soul. This heritage, passed down through generations, shaped her childhood and sparked a deep passion for natural medicine–a passion that would eventually become the guiding force of her life.

The journey, however, was not without obstacles. In her youth, Isabel faced a period of profound difficulty: after her separation, she embraced the sole responsibility of raising her daughters. These were challenging times, with motherhood pushing her to her limits while simultaneously fueling her determination to persevere. Even during moments of uncertainty, she remained steadfast, drawing strength from her unwavering commitment to her values and her profound connection to natural health, which always served as her refuge and inspiration.

Rather than yielding to adversity, Isabel channeled it into a drive for learning and growth. She dedicated countless hours to studying books on medicinal plants, exploring new healing methods, and deepening her knowledge of natural remedies. Over the years, she pursued extensive training in naturopathy, nutrition, and complementary therapies, often sacrificing personal comforts to follow her passion. Her dedication not only provided for her family but also enabled her to profoundly impact the lives of those who sought her guidance. People came to trust her wisdom, turning to her for advice and support, and her efforts ignited transformations in countless lives.

A pivotal moment came in the 1990s when she made the decision to professionalize her calling. She embarked on formal training as a naturopath and therapist specializing in alternative health practices. This step was transformative, opening new doors and broadening her ability to serve others. Her expertise, combined with her authentic desire to help, allowed her to support a growing community of people. Every story of healing and recovery deepened her sense of purpose, and she rebuilt her life around her mission to uplift others.

But Isabel's hunger for knowledge and her desire to inspire others extended beyond her immediate community. In 2017, she took a bold new step: she began to write with the aim of sharing her hard-earned experiences and knowledge on a larger scale. Her books, written in an accessible and heartfelt style, are both informative and empowering. They seamlessly blend practical advice, recipes, and natural health alternatives, inspiring readers to embrace healthier, more balanced lifestyles. Every page radiates her warmth and passion, inviting readers to find solutions for their well-being from within and aligning them to the wisdom of nature.

Today, Isabel's work resonates with countless individuals, especially those seeking to regain their health or reconnect with a more intentional way of living. Her story stands as a powerful reminder that even the greatest challenges can lead to profound purpose. Through resilience and perseverance, she has not only transformed her own life but also paved the way for others to rediscover their harmony with nature and with themselves. Her legacy serves as a celebration of living in balance with the natural world and honoring the deep, inherent connection between humanity and the Earth—a testament that obstacles can be the stepping stones to new horizons and an invitation to care for our body, mind, and planet with respect, awareness, and love.

BIBLIOGRAPHY & SCIENTIFIC STUDIES

1. "Plantas Medicinales: El Dioscórides Renovado" - Pío Font Quer

2. "The Green Pharmacy: New Discoveries in Herbal Remedies for Common Diseases and Conditions from the World's Foremost Authority on Healing Herbs" - James A. Duke

3. "Healing Spices: How to Use 50 Everyday and Exotic Spices to Boost Health and Beat Disease" - Bharat B. Aggarwal

4. "Medicina Natural al Alcance de Todos" - Manuel Lezaeta Acharán

5. "The Complete Guide to Herbal Medicines" - Charles W. Fetrow y Juan R. Avila

6. "Herbal Medicine: Biomolecular and Clinical Aspects" - Iris F. F. Benzie y Sissi Wachtel-Galor

7. "Encyclopedia of Herbal Medicine" - Andrew Chevallier

8. "La Farmacia Natural" - Adriana Ortemberg

9. "Plantas Medicinales de Uso Común en México" - Enrique Bátiz Vázquez

10. "The Complete Illustrated Holistic Herbal: A Safe and Practical Guide to Making and Using Herbal Remedies" - David Hoffmann

11. "Herbal Remedies for Dummies" - Christopher Hobbs

12. "Adaptogens: Herbs for Strength, Stamina, and Stress Relief" - David Winston and Steven Maimes

13. "The New Healing Herbs: The Essential Guide to More Than 130 of Nature's Most Potent Herbal Remedies" - Michael Castleman

14. "Guía Práctica de las Plantas Medicinales" - Josep Lluís Berdonces i Serra

15. "Herbs for Hypertension: A Guide to Lowering High Blood Pressure Naturally" - John Lust

16. "Medicinal Plants of the World" - Ben-Erik van Wyk and Michael Wink

17. "Plantas Medicinales y Curativas" - Jorge D. Pamplona Roger

18. "The Herbal Drugstore: The Best Natural Alternatives to Over-the-Counter and Prescription Medicines" - Linda B. White and Steven Foster

19. "The Modern Herbal Dispensatory: A Medicine-Making Guide" - Thomas Easley and Steven Horne

20. "Healing Herbs: A Beginner's Guide to Identifying, Foraging, and Using Medicinal Plants" - Tina Sams

SCIENTIFIC STUDIES

1. "Coenzyme Q10 and Hypertension: A Review of the Clinical Data" - Frank M. Rosenfeldt, I. E. Haas, F. E. Krum, T. E. Rowland, G. E. Walker, T. W. Esmore

2. "The Effect of Coenzyme Q10 on Blood Pressure: A Meta-Analysis of Randomized Controlled Trials" - Rosenfeldt, F. L., Haas, S. J., Krum, H., Hadj, A., Ng, K., Watts, G. F.

3. "Coenzyme Q10: A Review of Its Promising Applications and Potential Adverse Effects" - Marcoff, L., Thompson, P. D.

4. "Effects of Oral L-Arginine on Blood Pressure: A Meta-Analysis of Randomized, Double-Blind, Placebo-Controlled Trials" - Lucotti, P., Setola, E., Monti, L. D., Galluccio, E., Costa, S., Sandoli, E., Fermo, I., Rabaiotti, G., Piatti, P.

5. "L-Arginine in the Management of Cardiovascular Diseases" - Böger, R. H.

6. "L-Arginine Supplementation and Blood Pressure: A Meta-Analysis of Randomized Controlled Trials" - Dong, J., Li, Y., Xu, H., Liu, S., Zhou, Q.

7. "The Effect of Magnesium Supplementation on Blood Pressure: A Meta-Analysis of Randomized Clinical Trials" - Jee, S. H., Miller, E. R., Guallar, E., Singh, V. K., Appel, L. J., Klag

8. "Magnesium Intake and Risk of Hypertension: A Meta-Analysis" - Song, Y., Wang, L., Pittas, A. G., Del Gobbo, L. C., Zhang, C., Manson, J. E., Hu, F. B.

9. "Effects of Magnesium Supplementation on Blood Pressure: A Meta-Analysis of Randomized Double-Blind Placebo-Controlled Trials" - Zhang, X., Li, Y., Del Gobbo, L. C., Rosanoff, A., Wang, J., Zhang, W., Song, Y.

10. "Omega-3 Fatty Acids and Blood Pressure: A Meta-Analysis of Randomized Controlled Trials" - Geleijnse, J. M., Giltay, E. J., Grobbee, D. E., Donders, A. R., Kok, F. J.

11. "Fish Oil Supplementation Reduces Blood Pressure and Systemic Vascular Resistance in Normotensive and Hypertensive Subjects" - Morris, M. C., Sacks, F., Rosner, B.

12. "Omega-3 Fatty Acids and Cardiovascular Disease: Effects on Risk Factors, Molecular Pathways, and Clinical Events" - Mozaffarian, D., Wu, J. H. Y.

13. "Potassium Intake, Stroke, and Cardiovascular Disease: A Meta-Analysis of Prospective Studies" - D'Elia, L., Barba, G., Cappuccio, F. P., Strazzullo, P.

14. "Effects of Increased Potassium Intake on Cardiovascular Risk Factors and Disease: A Systematic Review and Meta-Analyses" - Aburto, N. J., Hanson, S., Gutierrez, H., Hooper, L., Elliott, P., Cappuccio, F. P.

15. "Dietary Potassium Intake and the Risk of Stroke in Women: A Prospective Study" - Ascherio, A., Rimm, E. B., Hernán, M. A., Giovannucci, E. L., Kawachi, I., Stampfer, M. J., Willett

16. "Vitamin C and Blood Pressure Reduction: A Meta-Analysis of Randomized Controlled Trials" - Juraschek, S. P., Guallar, E., Appel, L. J., Miller, E. R.

17. "The Effect of Vitamin C Supplementation on Blood Pressure: A Randomized Controlled Trial" - Duffy, S. J., Gokce, N., Holbrook, M., Huang, A., Frei, B., Keaney, J. F., Vita, J. A.

18. "Vitamin C Supplementation in the Control of Hypertension" - Fotherby, M. D., Williams, J. C., Forster, L. A., Craner, P., Ferns

19. "Vitamin D and Hypertension: A Systematic Review and Meta-Analysis" - Kunutsor, S. K., Burgess, S., Munroe, P. B., Khan, H.

20. "The Role of Vitamin D in Blood Pressure Regulation: A Review" - Vaidya, A., Forman, J. P.

21. "Vitamin D and Cardiovascular Disease: A Systematic Review of the Evidence" - Wang, L., Manson, J. E., Song, Y., Sesso, H. D.

22. "Chicory Extracts as Antihypertensive Agents in Rats" - Abdel-Hameed, E. S., Bazaid, S. A., Sabra, A. N., El-Sayed, M. M.

23. "Antihypertensive Effects of Cichorium intybus Root Extract in Spontaneously Hypertensive Rats" - Pushparaj, P. N., Tan, C. H., Tan, B. K.

24. "Antioxidant and Antihypertensive Activities of Chicory (Cichorium intybus) Root Extract" - Ahmed, B., Al-Howiriny, T. A., Siddiqui, A. B.

25. "Cinnamon Intake Lowers Blood Pressure in Humans: A Review of Controlled Trials" - Akilen, R., Pimlott, Z., Tsiami, A.,

Robinson, N.

26. "The Effect of Cinnamon on Blood Pressure: A Meta-Analysis" - Allen, R. W., Schwartzman, E., Baker, W. L., Coleman, C. I., Phung, O. J.

27. "Cinnamon and Health: A Systematic Review of Preclinical and Clinical Studies" - Ranasinghe, P., Pigera, S., Premakumara, G. A., Galappaththy, P., Constantine, G. R., Katulanda, P.

28. "Horsetail (Equisetum arvense) as a Diuretic and Antihypertensive Agent" - Veit, M., Geiss, M., Kiesewetter, H.

29. "Antihypertensive and Diuretic Effects of Equisetum arvense in Rats" - Srivastava, S. K., Srivastava, S. K., Srivastava, S. D.

30. "Evaluation of Diuretic and Antihypertensive Activity of Equisetum arvense L. in Rats" - Ivanova, S., Mikhova, B., Najdenski, H., Tsvetkova, I., Kostova, I.

31. "Dandelion (Taraxacum officinale) Leaf Extract as a Diuretic and Antihypertensive Agent" - Clare, B. A., Conroy, R. S., Spelman

32. "The Diuretic and Antihypertensive Activity of Taraxacum officinale in a Rat Model" - Rácz-Kotilla, E., Rácz, G., Solomon, A.

33. "A Review of the Diuretic and Antihypertensive Effects of Dandelion" - Schutz, K., Carle, R., Schieber, A.

34. "Hawthorn (Crataegus spp.) in the Treatment of Cardiovascular Disease" - Pittler, M. H., Schmidt, K., Ernst, E.

35. "The Efficacy of Hawthorn Extract in the Treatment of Hypertension: A Review" - Tassell, M. C., Kingston, R., Gilroy, D., Lehane, M., Furey, A.

36. "Hawthorn: An Overview of the Research and Clinical Indications" - Asher, G. N., Corbett, A. H., Hawke, R. L.

37. "The Effect of Lavender on Blood Pressure: A Systematic Review and Meta-Analysis" - Hajhashemi, V., Ghannadi, A., Sharif, B.

38. "Lavender Aromatherapy in the Management of Hypertension: A Randomized Controlled Trial" - Conrad, P., Adams, C.

39. "Lavender and Its Therapeutic Effects on Blood Pressure: An Overview of the Literature" - Cavanagh, H. M. A., Wilkinson, J. M.

40. "Melissa officinalis Extracts and Their Antihypertensive Activity: An Overview" - Shakeri, A., Sahebkar, A., Javadi, B.

41. "Antihypertensive Effects of Lemon Balm (Melissa officinalis)

in Animal Models" - Kennedy, D. O., Wake, G., Savelev, S., Tildesley, N. T., Perry, E. K., Wesnes, K. A., Scholey, A. B.

42. "Therapeutic Effects of Melissa officinalis in Cardiovascular Disease: A Review" - Miroddi, M., Navarra, M., Quattropani, M. C., Calapai, G., Gangemi, S.

43. "Mistletoe (Viscum album) as an Antihypertensive Agent: A Review of the Literature" - Hajtó, T., Fodor, K., Perjési, P., Németh, P.

44. "The Cardiovascular Effects of Mistletoe: A Review and Meta-Analysis" - Büssing, A., Schietzel, M., Girke, M.

45. "Viscum album Extracts in the Treatment of Hypertension: An Overview of Clinical Trials" - Kienle, G. S., Kiene, H.

46. "Olive (Olea europaea) Leaf Extract and Its Antihypertensive Effects: A Review" - Lockyer, S., Rowland, I., Spencer, J. P. E., Yaqoob, P., Stonehouse, W.

47. "Antihypertensive Properties of Olive Leaf Extract in Human Subjects" - Susalit, E., Agus, N., Effendi, I., Tjandrawinata, R. R., Nofiarny, D., Perrinjaquet-Moccetti, T., Verbruggen, M.

48. "Olive Leaf Extract as a Potential Natural Antihypertensive Treatment: A Review of Clinical Trials" - Perrinjaquet-Moccetti, T., Busjahn, A., Schmidlin, C., Schmidt, A., Bradl, B., Aydogan

49. "Passionflower (Passiflora incarnata) in the Treatment of Hypertension: A Review" - Dhawan, K., Dhawan, S., Sharma, A.

50. "The Antihypertensive Effects of Passiflora incarnata: A Systematic Review" - Appel, K., Rose, T., Fiebich, B., Kammler, T., Hoffmann, C., Weiss, G., Gericke, N.

51. "Passiflora incarnata: An Overview of Its Antihypertensive and Cardiovascular Effects" - Soulimani, R., Younos, C., Jarmouni, S., Bousta, D., Misslin, R., Mortier, F.

52. "Valerian (Valeriana officinalis) and Its Effects on Blood Pressure: A Review" - Andreatini, R., Sartori, V. A., Seabra, M. L., Leite, J. R.

53. "The Role of Valerian in the Management of Hypertension: A Systematic Review" - Cropley, M., Cave, Z., Ellis, J., Middleton

54. "Valeriana officinalis: A Comprehensive Review of Its Antihypertensive Properties" - Bent, S., Padula, A., Moore, D., Patterson, M., Mehling, W.

55. "The Effects of Hibiscus sabdariffa on Blood Pressure: A Systematic Review and Meta-Analysis" - Hopkins, A. L., Lamm, M. G., Funk, J. L., Ritenbaugh, C.

56. "Antihypertensive Properties of Hibiscus sabdariffa: An Overview of Clinical and Preclinical Studies" - McKay, D. L., Chen, C. Y. O., Saltzman, E., Blumberg, J. B.

57. "The Efficacy of Hibiscus sabdariffa in the Management of Hypertension: A Review of Randomized Controlled Trials" - Odigie, I. P., Ettarh, R. R., Adigun, S. A.

58. "Garlic (Allium sativum) and Blood Pressure: A Meta-Analysis of Randomized Controlled Trials" - Ried, K., Frank, O. R., Stocks, N. P., Fakler, P., Sullivan, T.

59. "The Role of Garlic in Cardiovascular Health: An Overview of the Evidence" - Banerjee, S. K., Maulik, S. K.

60. "Garlic as an Antihypertensive Agent: A Review of the Clinical Evidence" - Reinhart, K. M., Talati, R., White, C. M., Coleman, C. I.

61. "Flaxseed Supplementation and Blood Pressure: A Systematic Review and Meta-Analysis" - Paschos, G. K., Magkos, F., Panagiotakos, D. B., Votteas, V., Zampelas, A.

62. "The Cardiovascular Benefits of Flaxseed: A Review of the Evidence" - Rodriguez-Leyva, D., Weighell, W., Edel, A. L., LaVallee, R., Dibrov, E., Pinneker, R., Guzman, R., Aliani, M., Pierce, G. N.

63. "Flaxseed and Its Effects on Blood Pressure: A Comprehensive Review" - Khalesi, S., Irwin, C., Schubert, M.

64. "Beetroot Juice and Blood Pressure: A Systematic Review and Meta-Analysis of Randomized Controlled Trials" - Siervo, M., Lara, J., Ogbonmwan, I., Mathers, J. C.

65. "The Antihypertensive Effects of Beetroot Juice: An Overview of Clinical Trials" - Hobbs, D. A., Kaffa, N., George, T. W., Methven, L., Lovegrove, J. A.

66. "Beetroot and Its Impact on Blood Pressure: A Review of the Evidence" - Coles, L. T., Clifton, P. M.

67. "Green Tea and Hypertension: A Meta-Analysis of Randomized Controlled Trials" - Peng, X., Zhou, R., Wang, B., Yu, X., Yang, X., Liu, K., Mi, M.

68. "The Effects of Green Tea on Blood Pressure: A Systematic Review" - Hodgson, J. M., Puddey, I. B., Burke, V., Beilin, L. J., Jordan, N.

69. "Green Tea and Cardiovascular Health: An Overview of the Benefits" - Kuriyama, S.

70. "Turmeric (Curcuma longa) and Its Potential Role in Blood Pressure Regulation: A Review" - Meng, S., Cao, J., Feng, Q., Peng,

J., Hu, Y.

71. "The Effects of Curcumin on Blood Pressure: A Systematic Review and Meta-Analysis of Randomized Controlled Trials" - Sahebkar, A., Serban, C., Ursoniu, S., Wong, N. D., Muntner, P., Graham, I. M., Mikhailidis, D. P., Rizzo, M., Lip, G. Y. H.

72. "Curcumin and Its Antihypertensive Properties: A Review of the Literature" - Panahi, Y., Khalili, N., Hosseini, M. S., Abbasinazari, M., Sahebkar, A.

COPYRIGHT & CREDITS	2
Prologue: A Guide to Wellness	3
INTRODUCTION	4
HYPERTENSION	6
Types of Hypertension	8
Causes	9
Symptoms of High Blood Pressure	12
Possible Long-Term Complications	14
Reduction of Symptoms and Prevention	16
Sports to Avoid with High Blood Pressure	19
Additional Remedies	20
How to Measure Blood Pressure Accurately	21
Diagnostic Medical Tests	22
Warning Signs	24
FREQUENTLY ASKED QUESTIONS	**27**
97 FAQs about Hypertension	27
SUGGESTED PRACTICAL PLAN	**41**
NUTRITIONAL SUPPLEMENTS	**44**
Essential Precautions	45
Nutritional Supplements and Hypertension	45
Coenzyme Q10	45
L-Arginine	46
Magnesium	47
Omega-3	49
Potassium	50
Vitamin C	51
Vitamin D	52
Adverse Effects, Contraindications, and Interactions	53
Coenzyme Q10	53
L-arginine	53
Magnesium	54
Omega-3	54
Potassium	54
Vitamin C	54
Vitamin D	55
FOODS THAT TRANSFORM	**56**
Understanding the Link Between Nutrition and Health	57
Cooking Techniques	59
Healing Foods According to TCM	60

Apple (Malus pumila)	60
Bean (Vicia faba)	60
Celery (Apium graveolens)	61
Corn (Zea mays)	61
Cucumber (Cucumis sativus)	61
Garlic (Allium sativum)	61
Grape (Vitis vinifera)	62
Groundnut (Arachis hypogea)	62
Kiwifruit (Actinidia chinensis)	62
Lemon (Citrus limon)	62
Melon (Cucumis melo)	63
Mung Bean (Phaseolus radiatus)	63
Onion (Allium cepa)	63
Pea (Pisum sativum)	63
Persimmon (Diospyros kaki)	63
Plantain (Musa paradisiaca)	64
Sesame (Sesamum indicum)	64
Spinach (Spinacia oleracea):	64
Sunflower (Helianthus annuus)	65
Sweet Potato (Ipomoea batatas)	65
Tropical Pineapple (Ananas comosus)	65
Soybeans (Glycine max)	66
Tomato (Lycopersicon esculentum)	66
Additional Remedies	66
Caffeine and Hypertension: Ally or Silent Enemy?	67
Beneficial Foods and Beverages	70
Foods and Beverages to Limit or Avoid	72
Healthy Substitutes to Reduce Salt Intake	73
Hypertension Support: Easy and Tasty Recipes	73
JUICES & SMOOTHIES	**85**
Juices: Unleash Their Power	86
Homemade vs. Commercial Juices	88
Advantages of Homemade Juices	90
Possible Adverse Effects	91
When to Take Them	92
Preparation Tips	92
Key Recommendations	93
Nutritious Juice Recipes for Hypertension	95
MEDICINAL PLANTS	**97**

Essential Information	99
Guidelines for Care with Herbal Remedies	99
Measurements	100
Medicinal Plants for Hypertension	100
Achicoria (Cichorium intybus)	101
Cinnamon (Cinnamomum verum)	101
Hawthorn (Crataegus oxyacantha)	101
Horsetail (Equisetum arvense)	101
Lavender (Lavandula angustifolia)	102
Mistletoe (Viscum album)	102
Olive Tree (Olea europaea)	102
Phytotherapy Recipes	103
Simple Steps to Make a Tincture for Hypertension	104
Learn Everything You Need to Know About the Plants	105
Chicory (Cichorium intybus)	105
Cinnamon (Cinnamomum verum)	107
Dandelion (Taraxacum officinale)	109
Hawthorn (Crataegus monogyna)	111
Horsetail (Equisetum arvense)	113
Lavender (Lavandula angustifolia)	117
Lemon Balm (Melissa officinalis)	119
Mistletoe (Viscum album)	121
Olive Tree (Olea europaea)	123
Passionflower (Passiflora incarnata)	125
Valerian (Valeriana officinalis)	127
FINAL NOTE	**131**
AUTHOR'S BOOKS	**132**
Roots that Inspire: From Obstacles to New Horizons	**133**
BIBLIOGRAPHY & SCIENTIFIC STUDIES	**135**

www.ingramcontent.com/pod-product-compliance
Lightning Source LLC
Chambersburg PA
CBHW071831210526
45479CB00001B/85